Certification Review For

Health Unit Coordinators

Second Edition

Myrna LaFleur-Brooks
Founding President, National Association of Health Unit Coordinators
Director, Health Services Management Program
Gateway Community College
Phoenix, Arizona

Elaine Tight Gillingham
Director, Health Unit Coordinator Department
Gateway Community College
Phoenix, Arizona

W.B. SAUNDERS COMPANY
A Division of Harcourt Brace & Company
Philadelphia London Toronto Montreal Sydney Tokyo

AF778622

W.B. SAUNDERS COMPANY
A Division of
Harcourt Brace & Company

The Curtis Center
Independence Square West
Philadelphia, Pennsylvania 19106

Library of Congress Cataloging-in-Publication Data

LaFleur-Brooks, Myrna.

Certification review for health unit coordinators / Myrna LaFleur-Brooks, Elaine Tight Gillingham.—2nd ed.
p. cm.

Rev. ed. of: Certification review for health unit coordinators. 1989.

ISBN 0–7216–5669–2

1. Hospital ward clerks. 2. Medical records. 3. Medicine--Terminology. I. Gillingham, Elaine Tight. II. LaFleur-Brooks, Myrna. Certification review for health unit coordinators. III. Title.
[DNLMM: 1. Personnel questions—examination questions. 2. Medical records—examination questions. WX 18 L164c 1995]

RA972.55.L323 1995 651.5'04261—dc20
DNLM/DLC 94–36656

Certification Review For Health Unit Coordinators, Second Edition 0–7216–5669–2

Copyright © 1995, 1989 by W.B. Saunders Company

All rights reserved. No part of this publication may be reproduced or transmitted in any form or by any means, electronic or mechanical, including photocopy, recording, or any information storage and retrieval system, without permission in writing from the publisher.

Printed in the United States of America

Last digit is the print number: 9 8 7 6 5 4 3 2 1

To my fellow founding members of NAHUC -
Kay Cox, Carolyn Hinken, Helga Hegge,
Estella Johnson, Connie Johnston,
Kathy Jordan (deceased), Velma Kerschner,
Jane Pedersen, and Winnie Starr (deceased).

Myrna LaFleur-Brooks

To all the HUCs, CHUCs & SHUCs
who have enriched my life and to
my husband who is my life.

Elaine Gillingham

PREFACE

The second edition of *The Certification Review Book for Health Unit Coordinators,* as in the first edition, is designed to be a self-assessment of knowledge and practice of health unit coordinating. The textbook is intended to be a study guide for the Third Edition of *Health Unit Coordinating*, LaFleur-Brooks, W.B. Saunders Company. Preparing to sit for a certification exam requires one to address a large volume of material. Using the self-assessment review book will assist you in determining what you already know and what you need to learn. This awareness should ease the preparation process and assist you in making the best use of your time.

The book consists of sample multiple choice test questions, similar in style to those used on the national exam. The questions correspond with the chapters of the companion text, *Health Unit Coordinating.* The correct answer for each question and the rationale for the answer are provided. Each answer is followed by a reference page number of the companion text which guides you to more information on the subject matter as needed.

The Second Edition has been expanded to include questions abou the latest changes in health care technology as well as the latest in unit coordinating practice. A final section has been added to this second edition which addresses employment related situation questions. This portion deals with employment situations and decision making not included in the *Health Unit Coordinating* Third Edition companion text.

If you are reading this you have probably already decided to sit for the certification exam for health unit coordinators. Certification is a systematic process which recognizes and publicly attests to a person's mastery of knowledge and achievement of skills in a particular specialty. It is a voluntary process. Over 15,000 health unit coordinators (unit secretaries) have become certified since 1983 when the first exam was offered by the National Association of Health Unit Coordinators.

Recertification is now available by retaking the NAHUC certification exam every 3 years or by accumulating 48 CMUS (continuing maintenance units) over a 3 year period. By recertifying you will show a continued competence to practice in the health unit coordinator field. For more information regarding recertification, call 612-641-8095.

As more demands are being placed on the health care industry, hiring professional certified employees will assist institutions in meeting production demands. Being certified in your field may very well expand your opportunity for employment, for mobility, and possibly for career advancement.

We compliment you on your decision to sit for the exam and wish you success in this endeavor.

Myrna LaFleur-Brooks
Elaine Gillingham

ACKNOWLEDGMENTS

I would like to recognize the many talented people who generously volunteered their time, energy, and expertise to the organization and development of the National Association of Health Unit Coordinators. Without them we would not have the option of becoming a Certified Health Unit Coordinator. Also, my appreciation to those who have served tirelessly on the NAHUC Certification Board to bring validity and credibility to the certification process. A special thanks to the professionals listed below who assisted with the editing of the book. And finally, I want to recognize all the health unit coordinators who had the courage to sit for the examination. You have all greatly contributed to the evolution of your profession.

List of reviewers

Judith Graham, CHUC
Certification Board - Co-Director
50 Joppa Road
Merrimack, NH 03054-3121
(603) 424-6987

Mickey Sperry, CHUC
Certification Board - Co-Director
1805 East Central
Spokane, WA 99207-3438
(509) 489-1297

Madeline Clark, CHUC
Education Board Director
24B Dexter Street
Derry, NH 03038
(603) 432-6352

Cecil Powell, CHUC
Accreditation Board - Director
5022 Shoshone Drive
Pensacola, FL 32507
(904) 492-5783

Donna Kuhns, CHUC
Regional Representative
1812 North 51st Street
Milwaukee, WI 53208-1742
(414) 774-6294

Myra Holloway
Pitt Community College
PO Drawer 7007
Greenville, NC 27835
(919) 321-4455 (wk)
(919) 355-3807

Spring 1994 Health Unit
Coordinator Students

To obtain information about the certification examination, or recertification contact:

NAHUC
ASI Processing Center
718 Arch Street
Philadelphia, PA 19106
(800) 274-8719

To obtain information about the health unit coordinating profession, contact:

National Association of Health Unit Coordinators
1821 University Avenue
Suite 155 South
St. Paul, MN 55104
(612) 641-895

TIPS FOR TEST TAKING

1. Preparation for the test is vital. Plan for quality study time, at a desk or where you feel comfortable. Choose a quiet place, perhaps with your choice of background music; an environment without interruptions.

2. The exam is an objective exam, sometimes referred to as a multiple choice exam. Each question has a stem, the main portion of the question, and four options that either complete the statement or answer the question. There is one correct answer and three plausible distractors. The distractors are not meant to trick you but may distract you from the the correct answer.

3. Read the stem and each option as if it were a separate true-false statement. Eliminate those options you have left. Look for choices that give complete information.

4. Read each stem carefully. Look for key words in the stem such as first, most important, left or right, not, except and so forth.

5. Read all options carefully before selecting the correct answer. Do not read more into question.

6. Sometimes the option that has the most words is correct. Item writers are aware of this and may try to avoid giving this as a clue.

7. The number or letter of the correct answer may be the same as the several preceding it. When choosing your answer do not be tempted to vary your answer for this reason.

8. An option may be chosen on an impulse and then on review the option is changed. Avoid this. Studies have shown that the first answer that comes to mind is usually right.

9. Do not spend more than a minute or two on a question. If you are having difficulty selecting an answer, not that you did not answer the question, move on to the next, and then return to the unanswered questions when you have completed the exam. Subsequent questions may give you clue to the correct answer.

10. Take time to read the test-taking directions, then follow them carefully. Failure to do so may result in your correct answer being scored by the machine as a wrong answer. If, for example, your pencil mark is not in the exact required space, the machine may read it as an incorrect answer. Check that each question number matches the answer number. Do not hesitate to ask questions if you do not know how to proceed.

Allways, Never, all, every, None These words are Rarely correct

11. Answer all questions because the scoring is the same whether you answer incorrectly or not at all, and you may select the correct answer.

12. Prepare yourself mentally for the exam. Try positive mental imagery. Imagine yourself taking the test with the confidence that you are selecting the correct answers. Imagine yourself receiving a passing score. Having positive thoughts about your ability to perform can effect your actual performance.

13. Get plenty of rest the night before the exam.

CONTENTS

Section I: Orientation to the Hospital

Section II: Nonclinical Management of the Nursing Unit

Section III: The Patient's Chart and Transcription of Doctor's Orders

Section IV: Health Unit Coordinator Procedures

CONTENTS

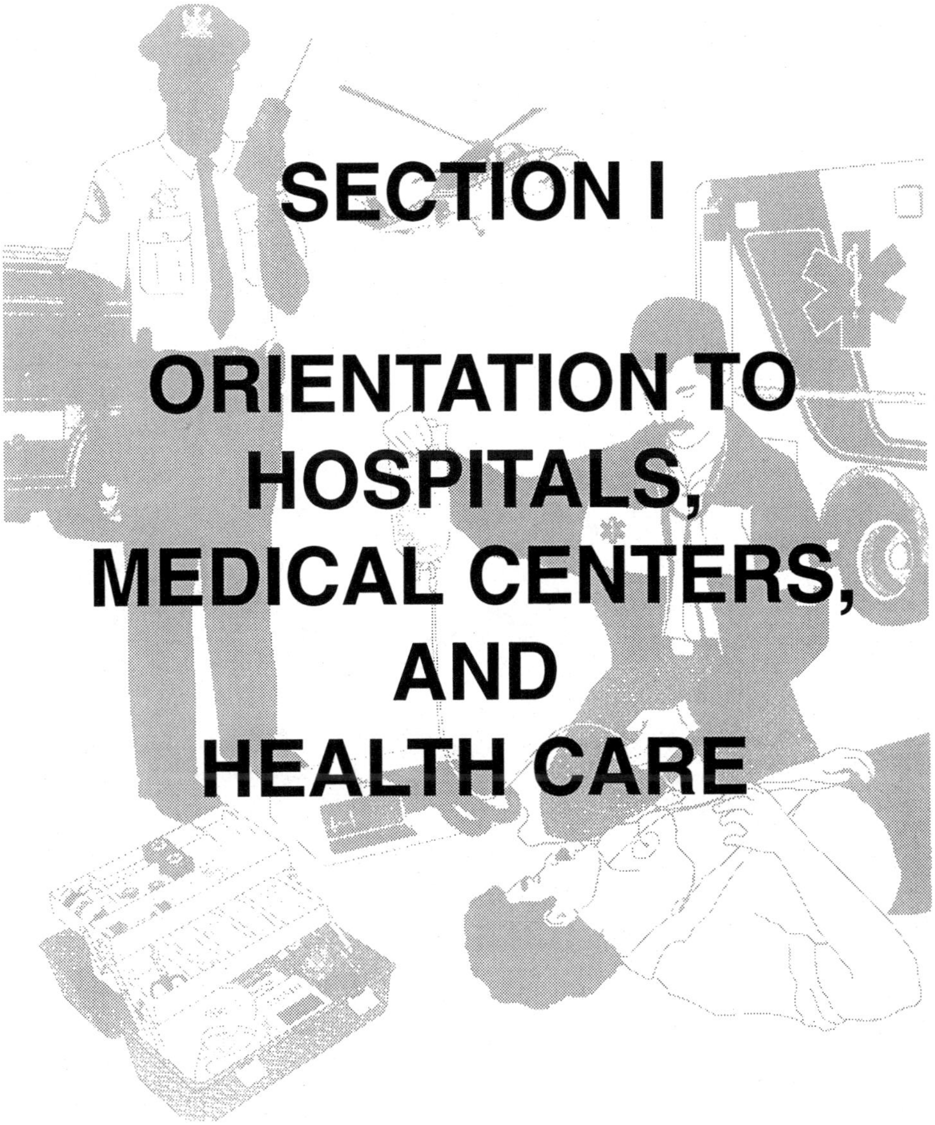

SECTION I

ORIENTATION TO HOSPITALS, MEDICAL CENTERS, AND HEALTH CARE

Chapter 1
Health Unit Coordinating: An Allied Health Career

1. Clinical tasks are performed at the:

   a. bedside
   b. clinic
   c. nurses' station
   d. doctors' office

2. Which of the following would not be a HUC task?

   a. scheduling a CT of the brain
   b. arranging transportation for a patient
   c. informing family members of test results
   d. calling a physician's office with lab results

3. Which of the following is licensed to practice medicine?

   a. registered nurse
   b. doctor
   c. pharmacist
   d. radiographer

4. A written process used to communicate doctors' orders to the nursing staff and other hospital departments is called:

   a. requisitioning
   b. transcription
   c. communication
   d. kardexing

5. The history of health unit coordinating can be traced to around:

   a. 1980
   b. 1960
   c. 1940
   d. 1920

6. Traditionally health professions, including health unit coordinating, evolve through four stages. Which of the following is not one of these stages?

   a. on the job training
   b. formal education
   c. formation of a union
   d. certification

7. National guidelines serving as a model of performance by which health unit coordinators shall conduct their actions are known as a:

   a. standard of practice
   b. code of ethics
   c. job description
   d. policy manual

8. Which of the following is considered a nonclinical task that the HUC may perform?

   a. placing a patient in the wheelchair
   b. serving the patient a food tray
   c. walking the patient in the hall
   d. answering a patient's call over the intercom

9. Dr. Smith is performing a L.P. procedure in the examining room. You hear a page for Dr. Smith and realize that the page cannot be heard in the exam room, your most appropriate action is to:

   a. ignore the page, knowing the operator will probably take the message
   b. ask the operator to transfer the call to the exam room
   c. explain to the operator that the doctor is busy and can be reached later
   d. take the message and deliver it to the doctor

ANSWERS AND RATIONALE

1. (a) Clinical tasks are performed at the bedside and involve providing direct care and treatment to or diagnostic procedures on the patient. p. 3.

> p3. refers to the page number in Health Unit Coordinating Third Edition, which is where you can find more information on the subject of the question. Using this text with the review book is a must in order to develop the knowledge base necessary for successfully completing the examination.

2. (c) Informing family members of test results is the responsibility of the physician or of the nurse. p. 6.

3. (b) The doctor (physician) is licensed to practice medicine. p. 1.

4. (b) The process is called transcription. Communication, requisitioning and kardexing are all parts of the process. p. 1.

5. (c) The first recorded use of health unit coordinators in the hospital was in 1940. p. 2.

> *The National Certification program is sponsored by the National Health Unit Coordinator Certification Board which is a part of the National Association of Health Unit Coordinators. The Association was established in 1980 in Phoenix, Arizona. The first certification examination was offered in 1983.*

6. (c) The third step is the formation of a professional association rather than a union. p. 2.

7. (a) The standard of practice is established by the professional association to be used as a standard nationwide. p. 4.

8. (d) Answering the patient s intercom is often the responsibility of the health unit coordinator. p. 10.

9. (d) Take the message and deliver it to the doctor. The HUC manages and performs the receptionist role for a nursing unit and performs the telephone communications for the nursing unit. p. 10.

> *L.P . is the abbreviation for lumbar puncture, a procedure used to remove cerebrospinal fluid from the spinal canal. See pp. 207 and 228.*

10. A transfer order is written and the physician requests a copy of the chart. You would follow the procedure as described in the:

a. HUC job description
b. health record guide
c. policy manual
d. PDR

11. To become certified as a health unit coordinator, an individual must:

a. pass the national certification exam
b. receive a certificate from an accredited school
c. be certified by the state department
d. pass a test sponsored by the employing hospital

12. The overall job of the health unit coordinator is to coordinate and perform:

a. clinical tasks for the nursing unit
b. nonclinical tasks for the nursing unit
c. all tasks requested by the head nurse
d. none of the above

13. Independent transcription may be described as:

a. the nurse caring for the patient is responsible for transcribing the physician's orders; cosignature not required
b. the HUC assumes full responsibility for transcription of physician's orders; cosignature by nurse in not required
c. the charge nurse transcribes the physician's orders; cosignature of the nurse caring for the patient is required
d. the HUC assumes full responsibility for the transcription of the physician's orders; cosignature of RN required

---

For information on joining NAHUC, The National Association for Health Unit Coordinators, or to obtain copies of the Standards of Practice and Education, or the Code of Ethics call (612)641-8095 or write to:

National Association of Health Unit Coordinators
1821 University Avenue, Suite 162 South
St. Paul, MN 55104-2869

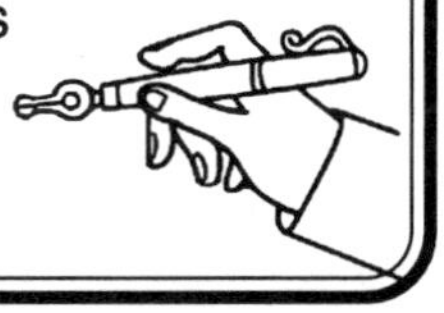

ANSWERS AND RATIONALE

10. (c) The policy manual contains guidelines for practice and hospital regulations. p. 1.

11. (a) A certified health unit coordinator or CHUC has passed the national health unit coordinator examination sponsored by the professional association, the National Association of Health Unit Coordinators. pp. 1, 3.

> Throughout this text the most up to date term "health unit coordinator" is used instead of unit secretary or ward clerk.

12. (b) The overall job of the health unit coordinator is to coordinate and perform the nonclinical tasks for the nursing unit. pp, 1, 4, 5.

13. (b) The HUC assumes full responsibility for transcription of doctors' order(s); therefore, cosignature by the nurse is not required. p. 1.

NOTES:

Chapter 2
The Nursing Department

1. The person responsible for patients and nursing personnel on a given nursing unit for 24 hours a day is called a:

   a. team leader
   b. nurse manager (head nurse)
   c. director of nursing (vice president of nursing)
   d. nursing supervisor

2. You are newly employed and find you need assistance with learning the procedures for your nursing unit. The department that is responsible for continuing education and that may assist you is called:

   a. staff development
   b. nursing service
   c. nursing unit administration
   d. personnel

3. A patient admitted to the hospital with the diagnosis of myocardial infarction would be admitted to the:

   a. DSU
   b. ICU
   c. MICU
   d. CCU

4. A patient entering the hospital for a cholecystectomy would be admitted to which of the following units?

   a. medical
   b. surgical
   c. gynecology
   d. urology

5. A patient entering the hospital with the diagnosis of Parkinson's disease would be admitted to which of the following units?

   a. behavioral health
   b. urology
   c. oncology
   d. neurology

6. A patient entering the hospital for a salpingo-oophorectomy would be admitted to which of the following units?

   a. gynecology
   b. neurology
   c. oncology
   d. urology

7. A patient entering the hospital with a compound fracture of the humerus would be admitted to which of the following units?

   a. medical
   b. oncology
   c. orthopedics
   d. rehabilitation

8. A patient entering the hospital for a TURP would be admitted to which of the following units?

   a. oncology
   b. neurology
   c. gynecology
   d. urology

9. Which of the following nursing personnel carry out the doctor s order to administer an IV medication?

   a. registered nurse
   b. monitor technician
   c. nursing assistant
   d. patient care technician

10. Which of the following nursing personnel would not administer Transderm-Nitro?

    a. CNA
    b. LPN
    c. RN
    d. LVN

ANSWERS AND RATIONALE

1. (b) The nurse manager (head nurse), is the person responsible for patients and nursing personnel on the nursing unit for 24 hours a day. pp. 14, 17.

> *Nurse manager is the current term for head nurse or and will be used throughout this text.*

2. (a) The staff development department, may also be called the education department, is responsible for continuing education. p. 14.

3. (d) The coronary care unit (CCU) cares for patients with heart disease such as myocardial infarction. pp. 14, 16, 17, 408.

4. (b) A cholecystectomy is a general surgical procedure; therefore the patient would be admitted to the surgical unit. pp. 16, 427.

5. (d) Parkinson's disease is a disease of the nervous system; therefore the patient would be admitted to the neurology unit. pp. 16, 388.

6. (a) Salpingo-oophorectomy is surgery on the female reproductive tract; therefore the patient would be admitted to the gynecology unit. pp. 16, 458.

7. (c) A fracture of the humerus involves the skeletal system; therefore the patient would be admitted to the orthopedic unit. pp. 16, 371, 373.

8. (d) A transurethral resection of the prostate (TURP) is surgery on the male reproductive tract; therefore the patient would be admitted to the urology unit. pp. 16, 445.

9. (a) The registered nurse would administer medications including IV medications. p. 17.

10. (a) Transderm-Nitro is a medication; therefore the certified nursing assistant (CNA) would not administer it. pp. 14, 17, 197.

> *CNA - certified nursing assistant*
> *LPN - licensed practical nurse*
> *RN - registered nurse*
> *LVN - licensed vocational nurse*

11. Team nursing method of patient care assignment is used on your nursing unit; you would communicate the message that the operating room is ready for Mr. Jones to the:

    a. team member
    b. team leader
    c. medication nurse
    d. nurse manager

12. Total patient care method of nursing care assignment is used on your nursing unit; you would communicate a patient discharge order to the:

    a. nurse in charge of the unit
    b. nurse caring for the patient
    c. licensed practical nurse
    d. team leader

13. An intensive care patient is improving and ready to leave the intensive care unit but needs more specialized care than is given on regular nursing unit. The patient would be transferred to:

    a. short stay unit
    b. recovery room
    c. step-down unit
    d. rehab.

14. A patient admitted with a diagnosis of PID would be admitted to:

    a. GYN
    b. ORTHO
    c. NEURO
    d. PACU

15. A patient having minor surgery but not requiring overnight hospitalization is admitted to which of the following?

    a. RR
    b. OR
    c. ER
    d. DSU

16. A patient is being admitted with a diagnosis of recurrent TIA, what unit would the patient be assigned to:

    a. ORTHO
    b. GYN
    c. CCU
    d. NEURO

17. A patient admitted with a epitheliocarcinoma would be admitted to:

    a. neurology
    b. oncology
    c. orthopedics
    d. rehabilitation

Test Taking Tip: **Preparation for the test is vital. Plan for quality study time, at a desk or where you feel comfortable. Choose a quiet place, perhaps with your choice of background music; an environment without interruptions.**

ANSWERS AND RATIONALE

11. (b) The team leader is notified of patient information by the health unit coordinator and s(he) in turn notifies the team members as needed. p. 230.

12. (b) The nurse caring for the patient is notified. pp. 23, 24.

13. (c) The patient would be transferred to a step-down unit where they would receive specialized care. p. 16.

> *Other terms used for step-down units are progressive care units and intermediate care units.*

14. (a) A pelvic inflammatory disease (PID) is any infection of the female pelvic organs, therefore, the patient would be admitted to the Gynecology (GYN) Unit. pp. 16, 454.

15. (d) Patients admitted for minor surgery but not requiring an overnight stay are admitted to the day surgery unit (DSU). pp. 14, 17.

16. (d) Transient Ischemic Attacks (TIA) are recurrent episodes of decreased neurologic function and would be admitted to the Neurology Unit. pp. 16, 387.

17. (b) Epitheliocarcinoma is a cancerous tumor composed of epithelial cells. The patient would be admitted to Oncology. pp. 16, 367.

NOTES:

Chapter 3
The Hospital Environment

1. The primary function of the hospital is:

   a. research of causes and treatment of disease
   b. disease prevention and patient education
   c. education of physicians and health care personnel
   d. care and treatment of the sick

2. Which of the following is not a way of classifying hospitals?

   a. type of patient service offered
   b. ownership of the hospital
   c. type of accreditation
   d. location of the hospital

3. Accreditation means that the hospital has:

   a. met an official standard
   b. a license to operate
   c. approval from the state department of health
   d. approval from a medical association

4. Which of the following departments of the hospital records and analyzes incidents that occur involving patients?

   a. security
   b. quality assurance
   c. human resources
   d. public relations

5. Which of the following is at the top of the organizational structure of the hospital?

   a. medical staff
   b. hospital CEO
   c. governing board
   d. advisory board

6. Which of the following is in direct charge of the hospital?

   a. medical staff
   b. chief executive officer
   c. governing board
   d. advisory board

7. Which of the following is not a responsibility of the governing board?

   a. establishing policies
   b. overseeing personnel standards
   c. supervising of quality care
   d. providing financing

8. A doctor wishing to join the medical staff of a hospital must be approved by the:

   a. medical staff
   b. governing board
   c. hospital CEO
   d. none of the above

9. The doctor who admits patients to the hospital is known as the:

   a. resident physician
   b. attending physician
   c. specialist physician
   d. intern physician

10. Which of the following is a medical school graduate gaining hospital experience?

    a. clinical clerk
    b. osteopath
    c. resident
    d. specialist

ANSWERS AND RATIONALE

1. (d) Options A, B and C are all functions of hospitals. Care and treatment of the sick is the primary function of the hospital. p. 24.

2. (d) Hospitals are not classified by their location. p. 30.

3. (a) Accreditation means the hospital has met an official standard such as accreditation from JCAHCO, the Joint Commission on Accreditation of Health Care Organizations. Accreditation is voluntary. A license to operate is required for a hospital to operate and is usually granted by the State Department of Health Services. pp. 24, 25.

4. (b) Quality assurance provides information to various departments within the hospital for the purpose of assisting those departments to provide quality care. p. 28.

5. (c) The governing board, also called the board of trustees or the board of directors, is at the top of the organizational structure. p. 25.

6. (b) The hospital chief executive officer (CEO) is in direct charge of the hospital and is responsible to the governing board. p. 25.

7. (c) The supervision of quality patient care is delegated by the board to a committee representative of the medical staff. p. 25.

8. (b) The governing board appoints doctors to the medical staff. p. 25.

9. (b) The attending physician admits the patient to the hospital. S/he may request a specialist to see and or treat the patient. p. 25.

10. (c) Resident is the term used to describe medical school graduates gaining hospital experience. p. 25.

NOTES:

11. The dietary department within the hospital is considered which of the following?

    a. support service
    b. diagnostic service
    c. therapeutic service
    d. operational service

12. You have just completed the order list for general supplies for the nursing unit, such as hospital forms and paper clips. To obtain the ordered items, you would forward the order list to the:

    a. business department
    b. purchasing department
    c. central service department
    d. transportation department

13. A radiologist is employed by which of the following hospital departments?

    a. cardiovascular studies
    b. electroencephalography
    c. diagnostic imaging
    c. respiratory care

14. Diagnostic studies related to brain wave disorders are performed in which of the following departments?

    a. neurodiagnostics
    b. endoscopy
    c. physical therapy
    d. diagnostic imaging

15. Personnel from which of the following departments assist in maintaining a patient on the ventilator?

    a. pulmonary function
    b. physical therapy
    c. respiratory care
    d. diagnostic imaging

16. The treatment of cancerous growths is carried out in which of the following departments?

    a. endoscopy
    b. pathology
    c. physical therapy
    d. radiation oncology

17. Upon discharge the patient's record is coded and then stored for future retrieval or for research. The department responsible for this is:

    a. personnel
    b. business office
    c. health records
    c. admitting

18. The hospital department that performs diagnostic procedures on body specimens, such as tissue, and also performs autopsies is:

    a. pulmonary function
    b. pathology
    c. endoscopy
    d. gastroenterology

19. The doctor's order for 1000 cc 5% D/W to run at 125 cc/hr add 20 mEq KCl is ordered from which of the following departments?

    a. central service
    b. dietary
    c. pharmacy
    d. pathology

ANSWERS AND RATIONALE

11. (c) The dietary department is considered a therapeutic service. p. 27.

12. (b) Unit supplies are ordered from the purchasing department, whereas the central service department stores and issues supplies used for patient care and treatment. p. 26.

13. (c) The radiologist, qualified in the use of x-ray and imaging devices, is employed by the diagnostic imaging department. p. 27.

14. (a) Diagnostic studies related to brain wave disorders are performed in the neurodiagnostics department. p. 28.

15. (c) Personnel from the respiratory care department assist in maintaining a patient on a ventilator. p. 28.

16. (d) Cancerous growths are treated in the radiation oncology department. p. 28.

17. (c) The health records department, also called medical records department, is responsible for coding, and storing records of discharged patients. p. 28.

18. (b) The pathology department performs diagnostic procedures on body specimens. p. 28.

19. (c) The IV solution is ordered from the pharmacy because it includes medication. p. 28.

NOTES:

20. A visitor is insisting, in a loud and angry voice, to see his wife. It is past visiting hours. You note the odor of alcohol on his breath. You are concerned that the visitor will become disruptive if his wishes are not met. You should call for assistance from which of the following departments?

a. administration
b. personnel
c. mechanical services
d. security

21. Which of the following conditions is treated by a gynecologist?

a. appendicitis
b. dysmenorrhea
c. dysentery
d. nephritis

22. An ophthalmologist treats which of the following conditions?

a. glaucoma
b. gastritis
c. aneurysm
d. emphysema

23. Disorders of the newborn are treated by a:

a. neurologist
b. neonatologist
c. geriatrist
d. gastroenterologist

24. Which of the following treats diseases of the aging?

a. pathologist
b. osteopath
c. geriatrist
d. gastroenterologist

25. Which of the following treats mental illness?

a. physiatrist
b. psychiatrist
c. neurologist
d. geriatrist

26. A family member informs you that he has obtained an attorney and is planning to sue the hospital for damages involving an incident that occurred involving his father while he was in the hospital. You should notify which of the following departments?

a. security
b. social services
c. risk management
d. public relations

27. An order for TPN should be sent to which of the following departments?

a. central service
b. laboratory
c. pharmacy
d. communications

28. An order for an EGD would be scheduled in which of the following departments?

a. gastroenterology
b. pulmonary
c. endoscopy
d. physical therapy

29. A patient with metastasis would be referred to which of the following specialists?

a. internist
b. ophthalmologist
c. orthopedist
d. oncologist

30. A "DO" is a:

a. director of obstetrics
b. doctor of osteopathy
c. doctor of orthopedics
d. directors of orthopedics

20. (d) Call the security department for assistance. You may also want to notify the nurse in charge. p. 29.

21. (b) A gynecologist treats disorders and diseases of the female reproductive tract. Dysmenorrhea is painful menstruation. pp. 27, 458.

22. (a) An ophthalmologist treats diseases and defects of the eye. Glaucoma is a disease caused by increased pressure within the eye. pp. 27, 402.

23. (b) A neonatologist treats disorders of the newborn. p. 27.

24. (c) A geriatrist treats diseases of the aging. p. 27.

25. (b) A psychiatrist diagnoses and treats mental illness. p. 27.

26. (c) Risk Management which may be part of the quality assurance department. p. 28.

> Risk Management, consisting of a variety of proactive efforts to prevent adverse events related to clinical care and facilities operations, is especially focused on avoiding medical malpractice.

27. (c) Total Parenteral Nutrition (TPN) or intravenous hyperalimentation is prepared in the pharmacy under sterile conditions. pp. 28, 187.

28. (c) The endoscopy department is responsible for performing diagnostic procedures by using endoscopes. An Esophagogastroduodenoscopy (EGD) is a visual inspection of the upper gastrointestinal tract. pp. 28. 253.

29. (d) An oncologist diagnoses and treats cancerous conditions. Metastasis is the transfer or spreading of disease from one organ or part of the body to another not directly connected with it. pp. 27, 362.

30. (b) A Doctor of Osteopathy (DO) places special emphasis on the relationship of organs and the musculoskeletal system. p. 25.

NOTES:

Chapter 4
Communication Devices and Their Uses

1. A list of options projected on the viewing screen of a computer is called:

   a. cursor
   b. menu
   c. keyboard
   d. data

2. The flashing symbol on a computer display screen that indicates the position where data may be entered is called the:

   a. password
   b. enter key
   c. cursor
   d. menu

3. Which of the following is the proper way to identify yourself when answering the telephone on the nursing unit?

   a. "First floor, may I help you?"
   b. "This is Suzie Que, first floor."
   c. "Suzie Que, Unit Coordinator, how may I help you?"
   d. "First floor, Suzie Que, Unit Coordinator."

4. When confronted with a question you cannot answer during a telephone conversation, a proper response is:

   a. "I'll get someone to answer the question for you."
   b. "I don't know, maybe the nurse does."
   c. "I don't know, do you want me to find out?"
   d. "Let me see if I can find someone to answer that for you."

5. Which of the following indicates proper telephone etiquette when placing a caller on hold?

   a. "Hang on, please."
   b. "Hold, please."
   c. "I'll place you on hold."
   d. "May I place you on hold?"

6. You have placed the caller on hold. To communicate this to the person who is receiving the call you should state the:

   a. name of the caller, nature of the call and incoming line
   b. name and nature of the call only; the incoming line will be flashing
   c. name of the caller and incoming line; the nature of the call can be determined later
   d. incoming line only

7. When requested by the nurse to place a call to the physician's office, you should plan first by recording the:

   a. patient's name, reason for the call and name of the person requesting the call
   b. patient's name, reason for the call, physician's office phone number and name of the person requesting the call
   c. patient's name, name of the person requesting the call, time, and physician's phone number
   d. none of the above

ANSWERS AND RATIONALE

1. (b) Menu is the name given to a list of options projected on the viewing screen. pp. 34, 38.

2. (c) The cursor indicates the position where data may be entered. pp. 34, 39.

> The view screen may also be called a monitor, a CRT (Cathode-Ray Tube), or a VDT (Video Display Terminal)

3. (d) Stating the nursing unit, your name and your status is the correct way to identify yourself when answering an incoming call. p. 35.

4. (a) A positive statement such as this will convey confidence over the phone to the caller. p. 35.

5. (d) Asking if you can place the caller on hold is the best customer relations approach. p. 35.

6. (a) Giving complete information allows for efficiency and good public relations. p. 35.

7. (b) Having this information at hand allows for the most efficient and effective use of your time. Recording the doctor's office number saves time should the call not be completed because of a busy number, interruptions, etc. p. 35. Skills Manual pp. 10, 11.

NOTES:

8. Which of the following should not be said over the intercom?

   a. "Mr. Butler, your wife, Scarlett, called; she will be in to see you at 7:00 tonight."
   b. "Miss Nightingale to the nurses station, please."
   c. "Yes, Mr. Butler, may I help you?"
   d. "Mr. Butler, I need to verify your weight, you are 250 lbs., right?"

9. A telecommunication device that transmits copies of written material over a telephone wire from one site to another is called a:

   a. fax machine
   b. computer
   c. pneumatic tube system
   d. pocket pager

10. You are giving "visiting information" to a father of a patient on your unit. You are the only employee at the nurses' station. The phone rings, you should:

    a. complete the conversation quickly then answer the phone
    b. excuse yourself from the conversation and answer the phone
    c. let the phone ring, they will call back
    d. continue with the conversation and pick up the phone while finishing the conversation

11. Which of the following is not a use of the computer on the nurses' station?

    a. to view stored information
    b. to process information for patient's admission
    c. to request diagnostic studies
    d. to print patient's bill

12. Notices placed on the bulletin board that require initialing to indicate they have been read should be:

    a. removed after a month and destroyed
    b. given to the nurse to be filed
    c. removed and placed on the nurse manager's desk
    d. sent to the nursing office

13. To contact a person by digital pager you would:

    a. call the operator with name of the person and a pager number for call back
    b. dial a pager number from a touch tone phone and dial a number for call back
    c. use the nursing unit intercom and verbally give a pager number for call back
    d. dial a pager number from a touch tone phone and verbally give a number for call back

---

Test Taking Tip: The exam is an objective exam, sometimes referred to as a multiple choice exam. Each question has a stem, the main portion of the question, and four options that either complete the statement or answer the question. There is one cone correct answer and three plausible distractors. The distractors are not meant to trick you but may distract you from the correct answer.

ANSWERS AND RATIONALE

8. (d) The patient's weight is confidential in nature. Confidential or sensitive information, such as weight, should not be communicated over the intercom. pp. 36, 47, 53.

9. (a) A fax machine is used to transmit patient information between departments within the hospital and from hospitals to other health care facilities or doctors' offices. pp. 34, 40.

10. (b) Answer the phone as soon as possible by excusing yourself from the conversation. pp. 34, 77.

11. (d) The hospital charges are determined by the business office. pp. 26, 38.

12. (c) Placing information that requires initialing on the desk for the nurse manager to review allows the follow-through needed. pp. 40, 41.

13. (b) To contact a person by digital pager, dial the pager number from a touch tone phone. Listen for a ring followed by a series of beeps. Dial your phone number followed by the pound sign (#). p. 37.

NOTES:

A voice pager is used in the same manner that a digital pager is used, except that after the series of beeps a verbal message is given.

SECTION II

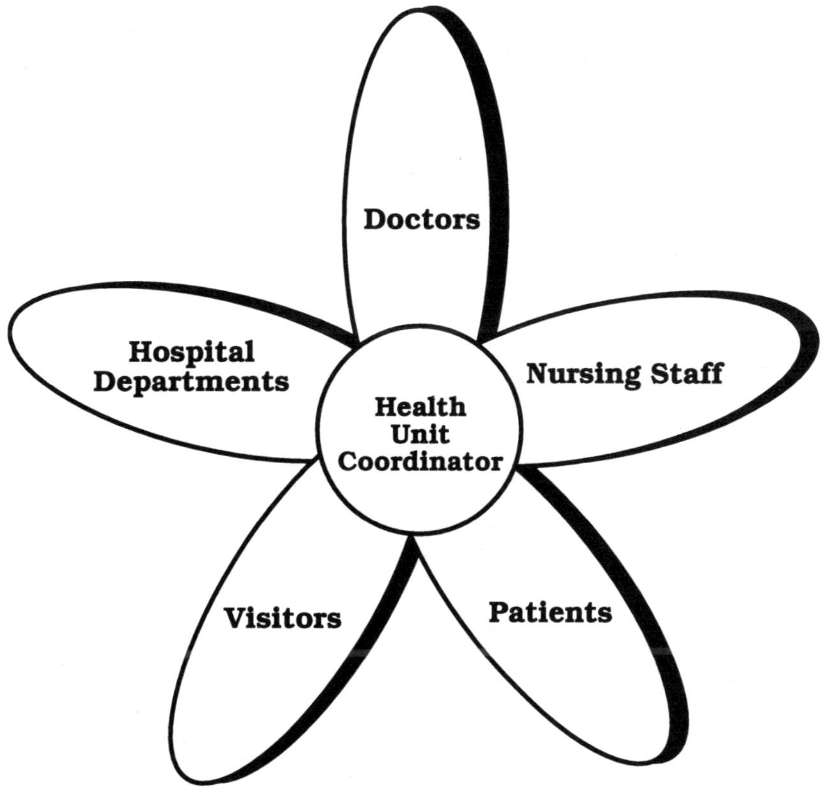

NONCLINICAL MANAGEMENT OF THE NURSING UNIT

Chapter 5
Communication and Interpersonal Skills for The Health Unit Coordinator

1. A respiratory therapist asks you if 423 bed 2 has an order for 0_2 to be started. Your best response would be:

   a. yes, he does
   b. check his chart
   c. give me the patient's name
   d. I don't know

2. A patient is brought by transport to your unit to be admitted. The nurse assigned to admit this patient is on a break. You would:

   a. ask the patient to wait at the desk until the nurse returns and prepare the chart
   b. escort the patient to her room and explain the use of the call light and the admitting routine and tell her the nurse will be there shortly
   c. direct the patient to her room, give her a book to read and tell her someone will be there shortly
   d. do nothing, your job is to assemble the chart and transcribe the doctor's orders

3. A patient's husband approaches the nursing station and states "Mary is in isolation! What for? I want to know exactly what is going on here." Your best response would be:

   a. ask the patient's nurse to answer his questions
   b. reassure him that this is sometimes necessary and there is really nothing to worry about
   c. tell him you don't know and have nothing to do with patients being placed in isolation
   d. advise him to put a call in to Mary's doctor

4. Which of the following is not a way to improve your listening skills?

   a. stop talking
   b. listen with your eyes
   c. suspend judgment
   d. think about how to respond

5. Which of the following is not a cause of ineffective communication?

   a. consistency between verbal and nonverbal messages
   b. poor listening habits
   c. poor choice of words
   d. inconsistency between verbal and nonverbal messages

6. When confronted with an angry telephone caller you should:

   a. put the caller on hold and locate the nurse manager to handle it
   b. hang up, since it is not your job to deal with such calls
   c. listen to the caller, acknowledge the anger and document what the caller is saying
   d. hand the phone receiver to the nearest nurse to handle

7. You have received a call from the local newspaper reporter who is inquiring about a celebrity admitted to your unit. You should:

   a. answer the reporter's questions
   b. refer the call to the patient
   c. refer the call to the charge nurse
   d. ask the patient if it is okay to answer the reporter's questions

ANSWERS AND RATIONALE

1. (c) Referring to patients by their room numbers may cause errors in treatment and care. pp. 48, 49.

> Referring to patients by their room numbers may interfere with esteem needs. See Maslow's Hierarchy of Needs. pp. 48, 49.

2. (b) Escort the patient to her room and explain the use of the call light and the admitting routine. p. 49.

> Explaining the hospital routine and patient expectations to a patient may help meet the patient's safety and security needs. See Maslow's Hierarcy of Needs. pp. 48, 49.

3. (c) Ask the patient's nurse to answer his questions. p. 49.

> The husband is concerned that he may contract what Mary has and he is concerned about her safety. See Maslow's Hierarchy of Needs. pp. 48, 49.

4. (d) Thinking of a response while someone is talking interferes with listening skills. p. 52.

5. (a) Consistency between verbal and nonverbal messages creates effective communication. pp. 51.

6. (c) Listen to the caller, acknowledge the anger and document what is being said. Do not become defensive. pp. 53.

7. (c) Refer the calls to the charge nurse. p. 54.

NOTES:

8. A friend of yours has been admitted to the hospital. You know that this friend has tested positive for HIV. You should notify:

   a. the friend's doctor
   b. the nurse manager
   c. no one
   d. the nurse caring for the friend

9. A visitor stops by the nursing station and remarks, "My friend Irma seems to be losing a lot of weight. How much does she weigh now?" An appropriate response would be:

   a. "That information is confidential."
   b. "That is really none of your business."
   c. "Let me look at her chart."
   d. "She is maintaining her weight."

10. A patient approaches you and says that she is afraid that she has cancer and that her doctor is keeping this information from her. You should:

   a. tell her not to worry, her doctor is competent
   b. find the correct information from her chart for her
   c. tell her she looks well, and everything will be okay
   d. tell her to share her concerns with the doctor

11. A fellow employee gave a presentation at a staff meeting and afterward shared with you that he felt he did poorly. An appropriate response would be:

   a. "I found your presentation very informative."
   b. "You were pretty nervous."
   c. "I've seen worse."
   d. "Maybe public speaking is not for you."

12. Another hospital employee approaches you in the cafeteria to ask the condition and diagnosis of her neighbor, who is a patient on your unit. You should:

   a. tell her to call you at home
   b. inform the employee that her neighbor may have visitors and suggest that she visit her
   c. since the person is a fellow employee, answer the questions
   d. pretend you don t know the answers

13. The sister of a patient calls the nursing unit and asks what diagnostic procedures have been ordered for her sister. An appropriate response is:

   a. refer the call to the nurse
   b. suggest that she contact her sister's physician
   c. ask her to call later
   d. tell her to ask her sister

14. You receive a call from a man identifying himself as a police officer. He requests a status report on a victim of a gang shooting. The patient has "NINP" written on his chart cover. You should:

   a. refer the call to the nurse manager
   b. hang up immediately
   c. transfer the call to the patient
   d. confirm the patient is on the unit but you can't give out any information

15. You are extremely busy, a doctor is insistent that you should stop what you are doing to get her a cup of coffee, your most appropriate response would be:

   a. I'm not paid to be a waitress
   b. get your own coffee
   c. I'll get your coffee in just a minute
   d. I'm very busy, the coffee and cups are in the report room, please help yourself

ANSWERS AND RATIONALE

8. (c) This information is confidential, notify no one. pp. 53, 54.

9. (a) Patient s weight is considered confidential information. pp. 53, 54.

10. (d) Suggesting the patient share her concerns with her physician is the best response. pp. 49, 65.

11. (a) "I found your presentation very informative" would give constructive feedback. p. 53.

12. (b) Inform the employee that her neighbor may have visitors and suggest that she visit her. You have the responsibility to maintain confidentiality of patient information. pp. 53, 54.

13. (a) Refer this call to the nurse, who will make the decision on what information can be shared with the sister. pp. 53, 54.

14. (a) No information, no publication (NINP) means that the unit denies having the patient and no information concerning the patient is to be given to anyone. The nurse manager will make the decision regarding the police officer. pp. 53, 54, 282.

> NINP may also be written as
>
> NE (non existent)

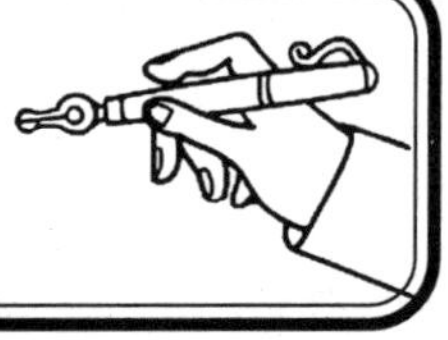

15. (d) Asking the doctor to help herself is an assertive response. A & B answers are aggressive and C answer is non assertive. p. 55.

NOTES:

16. You notice a visitor smoking in a patient's room where smoking is prohibited. An appropriate way of handling this situation would be for you to say:

    a. "Smoking is not allowed in the hospital, you may go outside if you wish to smoke."
    b. "I'm sorry but, smoking is not allowed but I won't report it just this once."
    c. "put out your cigarette, can't you see the no-smoking signs?"
    d. "put your cigarette out or I'll call security."

17. Dr. Seemore arrives on the nursing unit and loudly advises you that his patient, Mr. Polyp was unable to have his sigmoidoscopy completed because the order for the fleets enemas was not transcribed by the HUC. Your most appropriate response would be:

    a. "My signature is not the only one on those orders, the nurse should have caught that error."
    b. "I'm so busy and I don t ever get any help around here!"
    c. "The order was missed. I apologize for the error. Can the sigmoidoscopy be rescheduled for tomorrow?"
    d. "I'm so sorry, I can be so careless and stupid sometimes."

18. Jean, the HUC that relieves you on a regular basis, has become silent to you, causing an uncomfortable working situation. You would:

    a. ignore the situation and hope that the problem will resolve itself
    b. report the situation to the nurse manager
    c. only speak to Jean when absolutely necessary
    d. ask Jean what the problem is and talk about it

19. The holiday schedule is posted and you see that you are scheduled to work more holidays than all the other HUC's on the unit. You would:

    a. say nothing and bring it up on your next evaluation
    b. ask the other HUC's to give up some of their holidays in a trade with your days scheduled to work
    c. do nothing because its not really important
    d. go to the staffing office and bring the problem to their attention

20. Pat, a staff nurse that you work with is condescending toward you and makes disparaging remarks in conversation with you. Pat expects you to leave what you are doing to run special errands for her. You would:

    a. meet with Pat and tell her how you feel about the way you are being treated
    b. refuse to run errands for Pat and ignore her disparaging remarks
    c. report Pat's behavior to the nurse manager
    d. tell Pat you are fed up with her behavior and refuse to talk to her unless absolutely necessary

ANSWERS AND RATIONALE

16. (a) Advising the visitors of the rules is the assertive way of handling the situation. B answer is non assertive and C & D are both aggressive statements. p. 55.

17. (c) Admitting the error and offering a solution is the assertive response. A & B answers are aggressive and D answer is non assertive. p. 55.

18. (d) Ask Jean what the problem is and talk about it. This is the assertive way of dealing with the situation. pp. 54, 55.

19. (d) Taking the problem to the staffing office would be the assertive way of solving the problem. It may have been an oversight. pp. 54, 55.

20. (a) The assertive way of dealing with this problem would be to meet with Pat and express your feelings. pp. 54, 55.

NOTES:

Chapter 6
Medical/Legal Considerations

1. Which of the following statements is helpful in avoiding personal liability while on the job?

   a. have your orders cosigned by the registered nurse
   b. function within the scope of your job description
   c. always ask the physician to read the orders to you
   d. ask the nurse caring for the patient to verify all orders

2. Which of the following is the legal doctrine that holds the hospital as well as the employee liable for negligence?

   a. respondeat superior
   b. standard of care
   c. statute of limitations
   d. tort

3. The person who brings a lawsuit against another is called a:

   a. tort
   b. statute
   c. plaintiff
   d. defendant

4. The person legally responsible for your acts while you are working as a health unit coordinator is:

   a. the charge nurse
   b. the hospital administrator
   c. yourself
   d. the nurse cosigning the orders

5. Which of the following is an example of negligence by a health unit coordinator?

   a. s/he did not do what the nurse requested
   b. s/he transcribed the physician's order incorrectly, resulting in a patient injury
   c. s/he failed to remind the patient's nurse of a previously ordered daily treatment
   d. s/he took longer breaks than entitled to

6. Informed consent means that the:

   a. surgery department has been informed and the procedure is scheduled
   b. surgery procedure to be done has been written as an order by the physician
   c. person signing the consent has been informed of the risks and characteristics of the procedure and understands them
   d. nurse responsible for obtaining the appropriate signature has been informed

7. Which of the following is involved when a situation occurs that is in conflict with your personal value system?

   a. ethics
   b. legalities
   c. negligence
   d. torts

ANSWERS AND RATIONALE

1. (b) Functioning within your job description is a must. p. 70.

2. (a) Respondeat superior, which means "let the master respond," holds the hospital as well as the employee liable for negligence. p. 68.

3. (c) The person who brings a lawsuit against another is called the plaintiff. p. 68.

4. (c) You are legally responsible for your acts while working as a health unit coordinator. p. 69.

5. (b) Incorrectly transcribing a physician's order is an example of negligence. p. 69.

6. (c) Person signing the consent has been informed of the risks and characteristics of the procedure and understands them. Informed consent is a mandatory prerequisite for any invasive procedure or surgery. p. 69.

7. (a) An ethical dilemma is a situation that presents a conflicting moral claim. p. 70.

NOTES:

8. Tort means:

a. a wrong against another person or his property which is not a crime, and for which the law provides a remedy
b. the period of time in which a plaintiff must bring a civil suit
c. the condition of being responsible either for damages resulting from an injurious act or discharging an obligation or debt
d. professional negligence of a health care professional

9. The nursing unit is understaffed. A nurse asked you to help her out by feeding a patient. Your job description does not provide for you to perform clinical tasks. You should:

a. ask the patient if s/he would mind
b. feed the patient as a favor to the nurse
c. refuse to feed the patient
d. check if other health unit coordinators in the hospital feed patients

10. Accountability can be defined as:

a. answerable for what you have done
b. values, rules of conduct
c. a law
d. professional negligence

11. A deposition is:

a. testimony of a witness
b. pretrial statement of a witness under oath
c. values, rules of conduct
d. monetary compensation

Test Taking Tip: Read the stem and each option as if it were a separate true-false statement. Eliminate those options you have left. Look for choices that give complete information.

ANSWERS AND RATIONALE

8. (a) A tort is a wrong which is not a crime. p. 68.

9. (c) Feeding the patient is a clinical task not included in your job description. Should something untoward were to happen, such as the patient choking, the respondeat superior doctrine may not apply. p. 70.

10. (a) Accountability is being answerable to someone for something you have done. p. 68.

11. (b) A deposition is a pretrial statement given by a witness under oath. p. 68.

NOTES:

Chapter 7
Management Techniques for Health Unit Coordinating

1. You have just arrived on the nursing unit. Which of the following tasks that need to be done would you do first?

   a. relay the message to the nurse that surgery is sending for his/her patient
   b. order a stat CBC
   c. obtain a lab result for the doctor
   d. transcribe a discharge order

2. You returned from coffee break at 10:00 AM. The following orders on different patient's charts need to be transcribed. Which order would you start with?

   a. SMA6 and CBC in AM
   b. discharge order
   c. reg diet
   d. PA & Lat chest x-ray

3. How can you best keep track of the whereabouts of a patient's chart?

   a. make a notation on the census sheet
   b. use a patient activity sheet
   c. jot information on a scratch pad
   d. use a memory sheet

4. You would use a memory sheet to:

   a. list the tasks you are unable to complete momentarily
   b. assist you to remember difficult procedures
   c. record "difficult to remember phone" and pager numbers
   d. list routine phone numbers

5. An angry visitor approaches the nursing station and complains to you that her mother has not had a bath for two days. The appropriate response is:

   a. refer the visitor to her mother's nurse immediately, no need to waste your time listening
   b. listen to the complaint then explain that patient care is not your responsibility
   c. advise the visitor to report the incident to her mother's physician, s/he will take care of it
   d. listen to the visitor, tell her you understand her complaint and then ask her to wait while you get her mother's nurse

6. It is 3:00 PM, and the nursing unit is understaffed. The nurses are attempting to finish charting before shift change. A patient close to the nurses' station is requesting assistance to use the bedside commode. His nurse requests that you help the patient. An appropriate response is:

   a. "I can see that you need help, but I cannot do clinical tasks. Can I assist you in another way?"
   b. "That's not part of my job."
   c. "I see no problem in helping, since the patient is so close."
   d. "Let me just call the charge nurse for permission to do that for you."

ANSWERS AND RATIONALE

1. (a) Relay the message to the nurse that surgery is sending for his/her patient. p. 77.

2. (b) Transcribe the discharge order first so that the clerical work can be processed. p. 77.

3. (b) Record the time the patient and/or patient's chart leaves the unit and the destination beside the patient's name on the patient activity sheet. pp. 75, 76.

4. (a) Tasks you are unable to complete momentarily should be recorded on the memory sheet. pp. 77, 78.

5. (d) Respond to the visitor's initial remarks by listening and showing that you care, and then refer her to the appropriate person for further assistance. p. 77.

6. (a) It is important to function within the boundaries of your job description. pp. 79, 80.

NOTES:

7. Which of the following would you record on the patient activity sheet?

   a. lab results
   b. no code
   c. physician's name
   d. patient diagnosis

8. You find that the nursing station could be more functional if the chart forms were located closer to the charts. You should:

   a. discuss the change with the nurse manager
   b. move the chart forms and listen for feedback
   c. take a poll to see if everyone is in agreement
   d. leave the chart forms where they are; they were placed there for a reason

9. You arrive on the nursing unit to find several charts out of the rack lying around the nursing unit. Which of the following should you do first?

   a. replace all charts to the rack and proceed to transcribe orders of the flagged charts
   b. check each chart for new orders and stats, return them to the rack, then proceed to transcribe them
   c. leave the charts as you found them
   d. take one chart at a time, transcribe the orders and return the chart to the rack when completed

10. Nursing unit personnel should record nursing unit items running low on the:

    a. supply needs list
    b. patient activity sheet
    c. memory sheet
    d. census

11. A visitor approaches the nurses' station and asks you if his father may have a piece of chocolate candy. You should first:

    a. refer the visitor to the father's nurse
    b. read through the father's orders on the chart
    c. check the father's diet on the patient s kardex
    d. ask the father if he has been eating candy

12. You observe a visitor entering an isolation patient's room without following proper procedure. You should:

    a. call the patient's nurse
    b. advise the visitor of the proper procedure
    c. ignore the situation since it is not your responsibility
    d. tell the visitor to read the signs

13. A very hostile visitor approaches the nursing station with the complaint that her daughter has been ignored and treated rudely by the CNA. You should:

    a. reprimand the CNA
    b. explain to the visitor that the CNA is overworked and that she didn't mean to be rude
    c. advise the visitor to take the complaint to her daughter's physician
    d. listen to the visitor's complaint, tell her you understand how she feels and then get the appropriate team leader.

14. You find the unit is getting very busy and you are out of admission charts. An appropriate action would be:

    a. skip lunch break and assemble more admission charts
    b. call another unit for help
    c. call the nurse manager for help
    d. ask a volunteer to assemble more admission charts

ANSWERS AND RATIONALE

7. (b) No code is information you may use during the shift. pp. 75, 76.

8. (a) Discuss your idea with the nurse manager first. p. 77.

9. (b) Always check all charts out of the rack for new orders. Busy doctors can easily forget to flag charts with new orders. p. 77.

10. (a) Needed items are to be recorded on a supply needs list. p. 73.

11. (c) Check the father's diet order on the kardex form. p. 76.

12. (b) It is the responsibility of the health unit coordinator to communicate patient information to visitors. p. 76.

13. (d) Listening and responding appropriately is the first step in handling a visitor's complaint. p. 77.

14. (d) Ask a volunteer to assemble more admission charts (if available). p. 79.

NOTES:

SECTION III

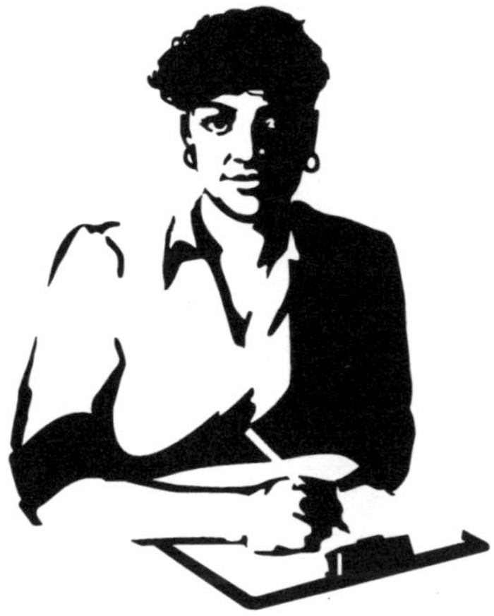

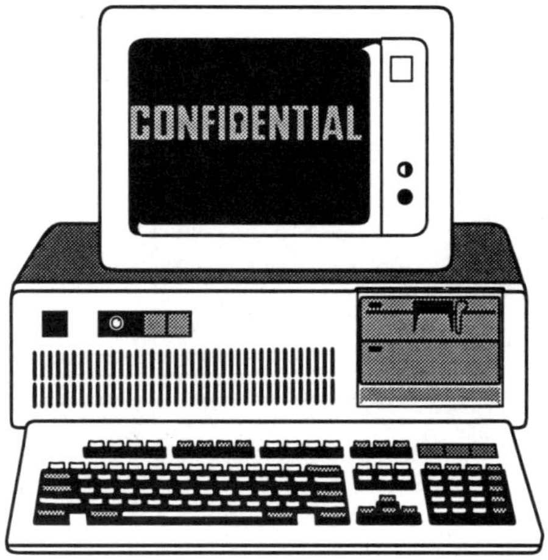

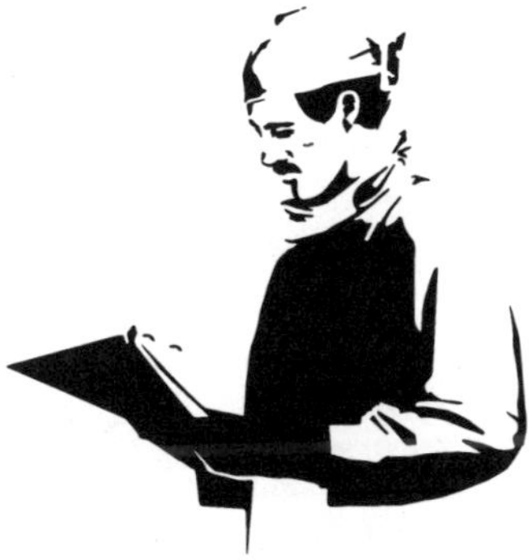

THE PATIENT'S CHART AND TRANSCRIPTION OF DOCTORS' ORDERS

Chapter 8
The Patient's Chart

1. Which of the following is a standard chart form?

    a. consent form
    b. anticoagulant record
    c. physician's order sheet
    d. diabetic record

2. Which of the following is a supplemental chart form?

    a. physician's order sheet
    b. progress record
    c. history and physical sheet
    d. consultation form

3. Which of the following is not a purpose of the patient's chart?

    a. means of communication between the physician and the patient
    b. planning patient care
    c. provides a written record of the patient's illness and treatment
    d. research and educational purposes

4. Upon discharge the patient's chart is sent to the:

    a. business office to determine charges
    b. physician's office to be available for follow-up care
    c. health record department to be stored
    d. home care department to be stored and/or used for home care

5. Which of the following is not a correct statement:

    a. all chart form entries must be made in ink
    b. written entries on chart forms must be legible and accurate
    c. errors recorded on the patient's chart may be obliterated and the correct information inserted
    d. written entries on the chart form must include the date and time

6. Twelve midnight in military time is:

    a. 1200
    b. 0120
    c. 0024
    d. 2400

7. Three-thirty in the afternoon in military time is:

    a. 0330
    b. 1630
    c. 1530
    d. 3300

8. A patient asks you to see his/her chart. An appropriate action would be:

    a. give the chart to the patient to review on the nursing unit under your supervision
    b. make a copy of the chart for the patient, since they have a right to their own chart
    c. tell the patient the chart is a legal document belonging to the hospital and he/she is not allowed to view it
    d. consult with the health record's medical/legal expert and with the patient's doctor

ANSWERS AND RATIONALE

1. (c) Standard chart forms are those commonly used on all patient's charts. A physician's order sheet is used to indicate care and treatment for a hospitalized patient. p. 89.

2. (d) Supplemental chart forms are used depending on the patient's care and treatment. The consultation form is considered a supplemental form. p. 97.

3. (a) The chart is not a means of communication between the physician and the patient but is a means of communication between the physician and hospital staff. p. 85.

4. (c) The discharged patient's chart is sent to the health record department where it is indexed and stored. pp. 85, 86.

5. (c) The chart is a legal document, errors cannot be obliterated. p. 86.

6. (d) 2400 is twelve midnight in military time. p. 86.

7. (c) 1530 is three-thirty P.M. in military time. p. 86.

8. (d) Consult with the medical/legal expert and the patient's doctor to assist you in handling this request. p. 86.

NOTES:

9. A patient receiving Coumadin would require which of the following forms placed on his/her chart?

   a. diabetic record
   b. clinical record
   c. anticoagulant therapy record
   d. respiratory care therapy record

10. A newly admitted patient's physician's order sheet has been imprinted with the wrong imprinter card. You should:

   a. discard the order sheet and ask the physician to rewrite the orders
   b. draw an X across incorrect information and imprint the correct information next to or below the error
   c. place a label over incorrect information and imprint with the correct information
   d. rewrite the orders and ask the nurse to sign them with the doctor's name and her/his own

11. A patient receiving an intravenous infusion will have which of the following forms placed on his/her chart?

   a. therapy record
   b. anticoagulant record
   c. diabetic record
   d. parenteral fluid record

12. Which of the following is the correct recording on a surgical consent form?

   a. lt hip arthroplasty
   b. lt hip arthoplasty
   c. left hip arthroplasty
   d. left hip arthoplasty

13. Which of the following does not need to be considered when a patient is asked to sign a surgery consent?

   a. the patient must not be under the influence of any "mind-clouding" medications
   b. the patient must be of legal age
   c. the patient must be mentally competent
   d. the patient must be hospitalized

14. Which of the following is not the health unit coordinator's responsibility for maintaining the patient's chart?

   a. keep the chart where it can be seen at all times
   b. know the identity of persons having access to the charts
   c. properly label the patient's chart
   d. frequently check the charts for new physician's orders

15. Which of the following forms would be signed by the patient on admission to serve as a financial agreement and would set forth the general services that the hospital will provide?

   a. face sheet
   b. condition of admission
   c. advance directives
   d. DRG sheet

ANSWERS AND RATIONALE

9. (c) Coumadin is an anticoagulant, so an anticoagulant therapy record would be required. pp. 97, 197.

10. (b) Draw an X through incorrect information and imprint with correct information next to or below error. p. 118.

> Chart forms (that have notations on them) that are imprinted with an incorrect imprinter card or with the wrong imprinter card or affixed with the wrong or incorrect label may not be destroyed. The correct information may be imprinted with the patient's imprinter card next to or below the error or affixed with the correct label. It is also permissible to print the information in ink by hand. After the correct information has been placed on the chart form, an X should be made across the incorrect information and "mistaken entry" written above the first line. The date, your first initial, your last name, and your status should appear next to the words mistaken entry.

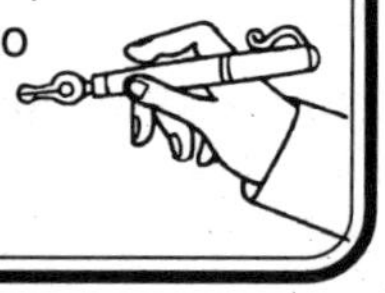

11. (d) The parenteral fluid sheet or infusion record is used by the nurse to record the types and amount of intravenous fluid administered to the patient. p. 107.

12. (c) Left hip arthroplasty is not abbreviated and is the correctly spelled procedure for a surgical consent form. pp. 111, 114, 115

13. (d) The patient does not need to be hospitalized to sign a consent form. pp. 115, 118.

14. (a) It is not necessary or possible to keep patient's charts where they can be seen at all times. p. 119.

15. (b) The condition of admission (C of A) would be signed on admission. pp. 91, 285, 286. (May also be called contract for services)

NOTES:

Chapter 9
Transcription of Doctor's Orders

1. A new set of doctor's orders can be recognized by the chart being:

   a. signed off
   b. in the rack
   c. flagged
   d. out of the rack

2. Which of the following is a "standing order"?

   a. MOM 30 cc po q6h as needed for constipation
   b. SSKI 3 mL in one glass of H_2O po qid
   c. Stat EKG $\overline{c}$ severe chest pain
   d. CXR PA and LAT in AM

3. Which of the following is a standing PRN order?

   a. Vistaril 50 mg IM q4h for N/V
   b. SMAC in AM
   c. Cefadyl 1 g IV q6h
   d. cimetidine 300 mg po at hs tonight

4. "Lomotil†- tab po qid until diarrhea subsides" is which of the following?

   a. standing or short order series
   b. PRN order
   c. one time or short order series
   d. stat order

5. The purpose of the kardex form is to:

   a. keep a record of patient information
   b. maintain a current profile of patient information
   c. order patient supplies and treatments
   d. keep the health unit coordinator updated on changes

6. Symbols are used in the transcription procedure to:

   a. indicate completion of each transcription step
   b. let the doctor know the orders are transcribed
   c. let the nurse know the orders are transcribed
   d. allow the nurse to evaluate the health unit coordinator

7. The process of recording data on the doctor's order sheet to indicate completion of transcription is called:

   a. flagging
   b. kardexing
   c. requisitioning
   d. signing-off

8. Symbols are recorded on the doctor's order sheet:

   a. after the transcription of all the orders
   b. before beginning each transcription step
   c. after finishing each transcription step
   d. none of the above

9. When in doubt about the interpretation of a doctor's order, you should:

   a. check with the patient to find out what the doctor told him/her
   b. avoid calling the doctor if possible, since this wastes his/her time and yours
   c. check with the registered nurse or doctor
   d. go with what you think, especially if it is a noncritical type of order

ANSWERS AND RATIONALE

1. (c) "Flagging" is the term used to describe the practice of identifying a patient's chart that has new doctor's orders recorded on the doctor's order sheet. p. 124.

2. (b) Standing orders are in effect until a discontinue or change order is written by the doctor. pp. 126, 191.

3. (a) The qualifying phrase for N/V (nausea and vomiting) makes this a PRN order and the order is executed according to the patient s needs. pp. 126, 191.

4. (a) This qualifying phrase "until diarrhea subsides", would make this is a standing or short order series. pp. 126, 191.

5. (b) The purpose of the kardex form is to maintain a current profile of patient information. pp. 124, 127.

6. (a) Symbols are used to indicate completion of each transcription step. Since transcribing, especially a long set of doctor's orders involves many steps and since the HUC is often interrupted, using symbols assists in avoiding errors of omission. p. 128.

7. (d) Signing-off indicates completion of transcription of a set of doctor's orders. pp. 124, 128.

8. (c) Symbols are recorded after completion of each step of transcription. If not done at this time the usefulness of using symbols is negated. pp. 124, 128.

9. (c) When in doubt about a doctor's order, always check with the doctor or the nurse. p. 138.

NOTES:

Chapter 10
Patient Activity, Patient Positioning, and Nursing Observation Orders

1. Pulse obtained at the wrist is called:

   a. radial pulse
   b. pulse rate
   c. apical pulse
   d. pedal pulse

2. I and O is the measurement of the patient's:

   a. food intake and output
   b. fluid intake and fluid output
   c. intravenous intake and urine output
   d. oral intake and urine output

3. Which of the following is a patient activity order?

   a. log roll
   b. wt daily
   c. NVS q2h
   d. OOB

4. Which of the following is the abbreviation for "every other day"?

   a. qd
   b. qod
   c. qid
   d. q24h

5. Which of the following is the abbreviation for "as desired"?

   a. as de
   b. ad lib
   c. as tol
   d. none of the above

6. "VS q4h" means taking:

   a. temperature, pulse, respiration and blood pressure four times a day
   b. temperature, pulse and respiration four times a day
   c. temperature, pulse and respiration every four hours
   d. temperature, pulse, respiration and blood pressure every four hours

7. Which of the following doctor's orders places the patient in a semi-sitting position?

   a. put patient in a Stryker frame
   b. may dangle
   c. Fowler's position
   d. none of the above

8. Which of the following indicates the patient is not to be out of bed?

   a. BRP
   b. CBR
   c. CBC
   d. OOB

9. Which of the following means "two times a day"?

   a. qid
   b. tid
   c. bid
   d. qd

10. Which of the following would be an appropriate order for a patient admitted with a contusion or heat trauma?

    a. CVP
    b. PCA
    c. NVS
    d. PAS

ANSWERS AND RATIONALE

1. (a) The radial pulse is obtained at the wrist. p. 142.

2. (b) Intake and output (I & O) is the measurement of the patient's total fluid intake, whether oral or intravenous, and the patient's fluid output. pp. 142, 146, 147.

3. (d) "OOB," or out of bed, is a patient activity order. pp. 142, 144.

4. (b) "qod" is the abbreviation for every other day. p. 142.

5. (b) "ad lib" is the abbreviation for "as desired." p. 256.

6. (d) "VS q4h" means taking temperature, pulse, respiration and blood pressure every four hours. pp. 142, 147.

7. (c) Fowler's position requires the patient to be placed in a semi-sitting position by elevating the head of the bed approximately 18 to 20 inches. pp. 142, 145.

8. (b) "CBR" is the abbreviation for complete bed rest; therefore the patient is not to be out of bed. pp. 142, 144.

9. (c) "bid" means two times a day. p. 142.

10. (c) Neurologic vital signs (NVS), the measurement of the function of the body's neurologic system; includes checking pupils of the eye, verbal response, and so forth. p. 142.

CVP - Central Venous Pressure

PCA - Patient-Controlled Analgesia

PAS - Pulsatile Antiembolism Stockings

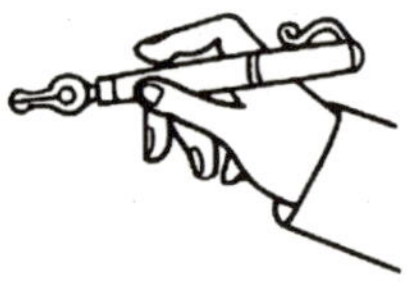

NOTES:

Chapter 11
Nursing Treatment Orders

1. The hospital department responsible for the distribution of supplies used for nursing procedures is:

   a. purchasing
   b. mechanical services
   c. business office
   d. central service

2. Reusable equipment should be promptly returned to the central service department to avoid:

   a. excessive patient charges
   b. contaminating other patients
   c. clutter in the utility room
   d. inaccurate inventory

3. When the nurse executes the order "TWE HS", (s)he will:

   a. insert a tube into the patient's urethra
   b. introduce fluid into the patient's rectum
   c. restrain the patient
   d. give the patient a bedtime snack

4. Colostomy irrigation is used to:

   a. remove stomach contents
   b. relieve gastric pressure
   c. wash out the urinary bladder
   d. regulate the discharge of stool

5. An indwelling or Foley catheter may also be referred to as:

   a. retention
   b. Hoffman
   c. nonretention
   d. residual

6. The order "cath for residual" requires the nurse to catheterize the patient:

   a. upon rising
   b. after voiding
   c. to determine patency
   d. after bladder irrigation

7. Which of the following is *not* a part of an intravenous therapy order?

   a. kind of solution
   b. rate of flow
   c. route of administration
   d. amount of solution

8. The doctor's order states the IV is to run at 100 cc/hr. You need to order the IV solution for the next 24 hr. How many 1000 cc bags would you order?

   a. one
   b. two
   c. three
   d. four

9. LR/5%D means:

   a. Lactated Ringer's with 5% distilled water
   b. Lacteal Ringer's with 5% dextrose
   c. Lactated Ringer's with 5% dextral
   d. Lactated Ringer's with 5% dextrose

10. The physician ordered an IV of 1000 cc of D5W @ 125 cc/hr. How many hours would it take to infuse?

    a. 8
    b. 10
    c. 12
    d. 14

ANSWERS AND RATIONALE

1. (d) The central service department (CSD) distributes the supplies used for nursing procedures (may also be referred to as SPD, supply purchasing department). p. 152.

2. (a) Patients are usually charged a rental fee for reusable equipment; therefore, promptly returning the equipment to central service after it is discontinued will avoid extra charges to the patient. pp. 152, 154.

3. (b) TWE is the abbreviation for tap water enema. An enema is the introduction of fluid into the rectum. pp. 151, 154, 155.

4. (d) A colostomy is an artificial opening into the colon which allows for the passage of stool. It acts as a substitute for the rectum and anus. Usually the rectum has been surgically removed. A colostomy irrigation regulates the discharge of stool through the colostomy. pp. 154, 155, 156, 426.

5. (a) A Foley catheter is a type of retention or indwelling catheter. The catheter remains in the bladder and is usually connected to a continuous drainage system. pp. 150, 156.

6. (b) Residual is the amount of urine remaining in the bladder after voiding; therefore, the patient is catheterized immediately after voiding to determine the amount of urine, if any, remaining in the bladder. p. 156.

7. (c) Route of administration is not part of an IV order since it is always administered intravenously. p. 157.

8. (c) To determine the number of bags needed, divide the amount in the bag by the amount of cc's to be administered per hour. 1000 cc / 100 cc = 10 hr. To cover 24 hours, three bags are needed. pp. 157, 158.

9. (d) LR/5%D means Lactated Ringer's with 5% dextrose. p. 158, Table 11-3.

10. (a) For the answer divide 1000 by 125. The correct answer is 8 hrs. pp. 157, 158.

NOTES:

11. The physician order reads 1000 cc of LR, @ 125 cc/hr x 3 days. How many 1000 cc bottles would need to be ordered to cover the three days?

    a. 9
    b. 10
    c. 11
    d. 12

12. Which of the following solutions is most commonly used along with administering blood?

    a. D/RL
    b. D/W
    c. NS
    d. LR

13. It is 2:00 PM. You have just returned to your unit from picking up blood from the Blood Bank. The nurse states that because of an emergency on the unit the blood will not be started during the shift which ends at 3:30 PM. You should:

    a. leave the blood on the desk with the requisition
    b. return the blood to the blood bank
    c. put the blood in the unit refrigerator
    d. place the blood with the patient's IV solutions

14. Which of the following is not a transfusion order?

    a. fresh frozen plasma
    b. cryoprecipitates
    c. LE cell prep
    d. plasma

15. An intermittent IV line is used for administering:

    a. all medications
    b. IV medications
    c. total parenteral nutrition
    d. tube feedings

16. A NG tube is connected to a(n):

    a. I-Med
    b. Emerson pump
    c. throat suction machine
    d. gastric suction machine

17. To transcribe the order "keep Hemovac compressed" you would:

    a. kardex the order and order the Hemovac
    b. check with the doctor for the amount of pressure
    c. kardex the order only
    d. order the Hemovac, a suction machine, and kardex the order

18. When ordering a "K-pad to upper left arm 15 min tid," you must include which of the following?

    a. number of K-pads
    b. heat setting
    c. size and shape
    d. disposable or reusable

19. Sitz bath is the application of warm water to the:

    a. feet
    b. pelvic area
    c. thoracic area
    d. whole body

11. (a) For the answer divide 1000 by 125, which tells you each bag will last 8 hours. Three days has a total of 72 hours. Divide 72 by 8, which tells you the total of bags needed for three days. The correct answer is 9 1000 cc bottles. pp. 157, 158.

12. (c) Normal saline is the most often used solution with the administration of blood. p. 159.

13. (b) The blood, if not given immediately, must be returned to the blood bank for storage, where safe, even temperature can be maintained. p. 159.

14. (c) LE cell prep is a laboratory test. p. 212.

15. (b) An intermittent IV line, also known as a heparin lock or buffalo cap, is used to administer IV medication to the patient when IV therapy is no longer needed. p. 158.

16. (d) The nasogastric (NG) or Levine tube is used to remove gastric contents. The tube is inserted through the nose into the stomach. p. 159.

17. (c) The Hemovac is a disposable wound-suction device usually placed in wound during surgery so you would kardex the order only. p. 160.

18. (c) K-pads are manufactured in different sizes and shapes designed to treat certain body parts. p. 161.

19. (b) Sitz bath is the application of warm water to the pelvic area. p. 162.

NOTES:

20. A foot cradle is used to:

a. prevent the top sheet from touching a body part
b. prevent footdrop
c. maintain a certain body position
d. apply heat to a certain body part

21. The doctors order for AE hose is a way for ordering:

a. hep lock
b. cutdown
c. elastic stockings
d. NG tube

22. When transcribing the order "OOB with elastic abd binder" you should include which of the following on the central service department requisition?

a. waist and hip measurement
b. chest and hip measurement
c. no measurement, one size fits all
d. height and weight

23. In the order "1000 cc 5% D/W KO," KO means:

a. add potassium
b. keep optional
c. keep open
d. knock off

24. An infusion pump or I-med is used to:

a. control the amount of IV fluid infused
b. drain fluid from the surgical site
c. insert the Foley catheter
d. irrigate the catheter

25. Which of the following orders would require a non retention catheter?

a. intermittent cath irrig 1 hr on 1 hr clamped
b. connect cath to continuous Hoffman irrig
c. cath for residual
d. irrig cath prn for patency

26. A small incision into the vein in order to insert a catheter for the purpose of administering IV fluid is called:

a. intracath
b. butterfly
c. cutdown
d. venipuncture

27. An electrical device used for applying continuous dry heat to the body is called a(n):

a. chux pad
b. K-pad
c. perineal pad
d. abdominal pad

28. To void means:

a. emptying the bladder
b. leaving a space on the kardex
c. emptying the bowel
d. emptying the stomach

29. In the order "change surgical dressings in AM" the order would be done:

a. this AM
b. tomorrow AM
c. every AM
d. anytime tomorrow

30. The order for TCDB would be entered in what area on the patient's kardex form:

a. vital signs
b. treatment
c. respiratory care
d. activity

20. (a) A foot cradle is a metal frame placed on the bed to prevent the top sheet from touching a specified part of the body. p. 163.

21. (c) AE (anti-embolism) hose are also called elastic stockings. pp. 163, 164.

> *T.E.D. is a brand name for elastic stockings. Order may specify one or both legs and thigh or knee high. Patient will need to be measured to insure correct fitting.*

22. (a) Usually the hip and waist measurements are necessary to obtain a correctly fitting binder. p. 163.

23. (c) KO means "keep open," or TKO "to keep open". When used in IV orders it is the rate of flow. IV rate is about 5cc/hr. p. 151.

24. (a) An infusion pump is used to control the amount of IV fluid. It is a reusable electric machine, obtained from the central service department. pp. 150, 158.

25. (c) A non retention catheter is used for residual. It is removed immediately following the procedure. p. 157.

26. (c) A cutdown is used when the patient has poor circulation, which makes venipuncture difficult. p. 157.

27. (b) A K-pad is used to apply continuous dry heat to the body. p. 161.

28. (a) Void means emptying the bladder. p.150.

29. (b) When used in writing doctor's orders, "this AM" means today and "in AM" means tomorrow. p. 150.

30. (b) Turn, cough, deep breathe (TCDB) is a nursing treatment order therefore is entered on the treatment area of the kardex form. p. 164.

NOTES:

31. The term given to blood that is donated for a patient by friends or relatives is:

   a. intraoperative blood cell salvage
   b. autologous blood
   c. donor-specific
   d. occult blood

32. An order reading Accu-Chek ac and hs means:

   a. check the glucose level of blood before meals and at bedtime
   b. check acquities before meals and at bedtime
   c. check the glucose level of blood after meals and at bedtime
   d. check acquities after meals and at bedtimes

33. An order reading "ORE today" means the patient is to have:

   a. overhead resistive exercises
   b. occupational rehabilitation exercises
   c. outpatient renal endoscopy
   d. oil retention enema

34. An order reading "insert Foley to st drain" means the nurse is to:

   a. insert a retention catheter to straight drainage
   b. insert a nonretention catheter to straight drainage
   c. insert a catheter to standard drain
   d. insert a non-retention catheter to obtain sterile drainage for specimen

35. The Jackson-Pratt is a/an:

   a. reusable wound-suction device
   b. electric device used for administering blood
   c. disposable wound-suction device
   d. electric device used for heat application

Test Taking Tip: **Read each stem carefully. Look for key words in the stem such as first, most important, left or right, not, except and so forth.**

31. (c) Donor specific or donor-directed blood is the term used for blood that is donated for a patient by relatives or friends prior to patient need. pp. 150, 159.

> ***Intraoperative Blood Cell Salvage*** *- patient's blood lost during surgery is transfused back into patient.*
>
> ***Autologous Blood*** *- the patient's own blood donated previously for transfusion as needed by the patient.*
>
> ***Occult Blood*** *- blood that is undetectable to the eye.*

32. (a) Accu-Chek is a type of commercial blood glucose monitor used to check the glucose level of blood; ac means before meals and hs means hours of sleep. pp. 151,165, 166.

33. (d) Oil retention enema (ORE) is a type of enema. pp. 151, 154.

34. (a) A Foley is a type of retention catheter and st is an abbreviation meaning straight. pp. 150, 151.

35. (c) The Jackson-Pratt is a disposable wound-suction device. p. 161.

NOTES:

Chapter 12
Dietary Orders

1. Feeding by means of a tube inserted into the stomach through an artificial opening in the abdominal wall is called:

   a. nasogastric feeding
   b. gavage feeding
   c. total parenteral nutrition
   d. gastrostomy feeding

2. Which of the following are considered special diets?

   1. soft
   2. modified fiber
   3. low cholesterol
   4. mechanical soft
   5. 4000 mg Na

      a. 1,2,3
      b. 2,3,5
      c. 2,3,4
      d. 3,4,5

3. Diet as tolerated includes which of the following choices?

   a. clear liquid, full liquid, soft, normal
   b. clear liquid, soft, normal, 2 gm Na
   c. full liquid, soft, normal, low fat
   d. none of the above

4. What would a physician's order for "DAT" require you to do?

   a. send an order to dietary for DAT
   b. check with the patient's nurse
   c. check with the patient
   d. ask the physician to clarify order

5. An order for "FF" means that:

   a. all food should be fast fried
   b. extra fluids should be given against patient's will
   c. an IV should be started
   d. extra fluids should be offered to the patient

6. The doctor's order for sips and chips means the patient may have:

   a. sips of water and ice chips
   b. carbonated water and ice chips
   c. Coke and potato chips
   d. tea and ice chips

7. Which of the following diets differ from the normal diet in consistency of the food?

   1. low sodium
   2. full liquid
   3. mechanical soft
   4. gluten-free
   5. high potassium

      a. 1 and 2
      b. 2 and 3
      c. 3 and 4
      d. 4 and 5

8. In the doctor's order "1000 cal ADA diet," ADA means:

   a. adjust down amount
   b. American Diabetic Association
   c. American Dietetic Association
   d. none of the above

ANSWERS AND RATIONALE

1. (d) Ensure, blenderized or standard formula are fed to the patient through a gastrostomy tube inserted through the abdominal wall into the stomach. pp. 170, 173.

2. (b) Modified fiber, low cholesterol, and 4000 mg Na (sodium) are special diets. Soft and mechanical soft are normal diets with consistency variations. pp. 172, 173.

3. (a) Clear liquid, full liquid, soft and normal are choices appropriate for diet as tolerated. p. 173.

4. (b) Diet as tolerated (DAT) would require you to check with the patient's nurse to determine the type of diet to order for the patient. pp. 170, 173.

5. (d) Force fluids (FF) means that extra fluids should be offered to the patient. pp. 170, 174.

6. (a) Sips and chips means the patient may have sips of water and ice chips. p. 175.

7. (b) Both full liquid and mechanical diets differ from a normal diet in consistency of the food. pp. 172, 173.

8. (b) ADA stands for the American Diabetic Association. p. 170.

NOTES:

9. In the order "Ensure Plus via bolus feeding 400 cc q6h." Bolus means:

   a. allows the formula to run in by gravity
   b. infuse a small amount of formula over a short time
   c. control the rate of administration
   d. is the name of the feeding tube

10. Which of the following is not a commercialized prepared formula?

   a. Osmolite
   b. Jevity
   c. Vivonex -Ten
   d. Dobbhoff

11. What would you order in transcribing the following doctor's order? "Insert Dobbhoff, x-ray for placement. When in proper position, begin via pump, Jevity 1/2 strength, dilute with H_2O TRA 400cc/h for 8h, then 50cc/h for 8h, then FS Jevity at 50cc/hr."

   a. feeding tube, x-ray, Jevity
   b. feeding tube, Imed, Jevity, x-ray
   c. feeding tube, feeding infusion pump, x-ray and Jevity
   d. Dobbhoff, Jevity and x-ray

Test Taking Tip: Read all options carefully before selecting the correct answer. Do not read more into the question.

ANSWERS AND RATIONALE

9. (b) Bolus consists of infusing a small amount of formula over a short time. p. 173.

10. (d) Dobbhoff is the name of a nasogastric tube (feeding). p. 173.

11. (c) Dobbhoff (a NG feeding tube), feeding infusionpump, x-ray and Jevity. p. 173.

NOTES:

Chapter 13
Medication Orders

1. Adding a medication to a container of intravenous solution is called:

   a. piggy-back
   b. suspension
   c. IV push
   d. admixture

2. A decimal system of weights and measures based on multiples of ten is called:

   a. ampule
   b. apothecary
   c. metric
   d. generic

3. A method by which drugs are administered intravenously in 50 to 100 milliliters of fluid is called:

   a. IV push
   b. IVPB
   c. intravenous hyperalimentation
   d. parenteral

4. A gelatinous container in which a drug is enclosed is called:

   a. ampule
   b. tablet
   c. suppository
   d. capsule

5. In which of the following orders is the solution injected under the skin into fat or connective tissue?

   a. Keflin 0.5 g IVPB q8h
   b. MS 10 mg IM q4h prn pain
   c. heparin 10,000 U sub-q stat
   d. Lanoxin 0.5 mg IV push

6. In the order "Garamycin ophth sol gtt i OS tid," the medication is to be administered in:

   a. the left eye
   b. both eyes
   c. the right eye
   d. none of the above

7. In the order "1000 mL 5% D/W @ KO rate," the mL means:

   a. milliequivalent
   b. milligram
   c. millimeter
   d. none of the above

8. In the order "Maalox 15 cc tid pc," pc means:

   a. before meals
   b. after meals
   c. as needed
   d. none of the above

9. A type of medication that relieves pain is called:

   a. narcotic
   b. tranquilizer
   c. hormone
   d. hypnotic

10. A shortened name given to a drug by a developer is the:

    a. official name
    b. chemical name
    c. generic name
    d. trade name

ANSWERS AND RATIONALE

1. (d) Admixture is the result of adding a medication to a container of IV solution. pp. 177, 187.

2. (c) The metric system is a system of weights and measures based on multiples of ten. pp. 185, 186.

3. (b) Intravenous piggy-back (IVPB) is a method of administering drugs intravenously in 50 to 100 milliliters of fluid. pp. 177, 189.

4. (d) A capsule is a gelatinous container in which a drug is enclosed. p. 177.

5. (c) Sub-q is the abbreviation for subcutaneous injection, which is the introduction of a medication under the skin into the fat or connective tissue. pp. 177, 186.

6. (a) OS is the abbreviation for left eye. p. 178.

7. (d) mL is the abbreviation for milliliter. p. 178.

8. (b) pc is the abbreviation for after meals. p. 178.

9. (a) A narcotic relieves pain and sometimes produces sleep. pp. 177, 193.

10. (c) Generic is the shortened name given to the drug by the developer so that the long chemical name need not be used. p. 183.

Generic names of drugs are not capitalized (meperidine). The brand name is always capitalized and may have a trademark symbol (Demerol).

NOTES:

11. Which component of a medication order is missing in the physician's order "Aspirin EC po q3h prn"?

   a. name of drug
   b. dosage of drug
   c. route of administration
   d. frequency of administration

12. The apothecary measurement grain iss means:

   a. one and one-quarter grains
   b. one and one-half grains
   c. one and one-eighth grains
   d. none of the above

13. Which of the following is *not* used to indicate a specific form of medication?

   a. capsule
   b. enteric-coated
   c. liter
   d. suppository

14. Which of the following is *not* a unit of the metric system?

   a. gram
   b. liter
   c. meter
   d. dram

15. Which of the following is a nutrition given through a central venous catheter?

   a. TPN
   b. IVPB
   c. IV
   d. PPD

16. Which of the following drugs is *not* a controlled substance?

   a. Demerol
   b. Seconal
   c. Mefoxin
   d. Doriden

17. 1000 cc is the same as:

   a. 1000 mg
   b. 1000 mL
   c. 1000 mEq
   d. 1000 L

18. Which of the following is a non-narcotic analgesic used to lessen pain?

   a. Dilantin
   b. Percodan
   c. Empirin
   d. Amphojel

19. Which of the following drugs may be ordered as a treatment for arthritis?

   a. Indocin
   b. Orinase
   c. Actifed
   d. Inderal

20. Which of the following drugs is a vasodilator which will lower blood pressure by relaxing the blood vessel walls?

   a. Tagamet
   b. Apresoline
   c. Compazine
   d. Lanoxin

21. Which of the following medications is an antianemic drug which would be given to build up iron in the blood?

   a. Fiorinal
   b. prednisone
   c. Imferon
   d. Tofranil

22. Which of the following is a diuretic?

   a. Lasix
   b. digoxin
   c. Cytoxan
   d. Adrenalin

ANSWERS AND RATIONALE

11. (b) The dosage of the drug is missing. pp. 183, 184.

12. (b) grain $\overline{\dot{\imath}\text{ss}}$ means one and one-half grains. p. 184.

13. (c) Liter indicates volume rather than form. pp. 185, 186.

14. (d) Dram is a term relating to volume (liquid) in the apothecary system. p. 184.

15. (a) TPN, total parenteral nutrition, or hyperalimentation is a nutrition given through a central venous catheter. pp. 177, 178, 187, 189.

16. (c) Mefoxin is an antibiotic. Antibiotics are not controlled substances although they usually have an automatic stop date. p. 194.

17. (b) The terms milliliter (mL) and cubic centimeter (cc) are used interchangeably. p. 185.

18. (c) Empirin is a non-narcotic analgesic. p. 194.

19. (a) Indocin is an antiarthritic drug ordered to reduce inflammation and relieve pain in arthritis or arthritis-like conditions. p. 196.

20. (b) Apresoline is a vasodilator which may be ordered to lower blood pressure. p. 197.

21. (c) Imferon is an antianemic drug. p. 195.

> *Antianemic drugs may often be recognized by the letters "fe" included in the name of the drug. Fe is the symbol for iron.*

22. (a) Lasix is a diuretic drug which stimulates the flow of urine. p. 196.

NOTES:

Cubic centermeters
Milliliters

23. Which of the following drugs is a tranquilizer?

a. Gantrisin
b. Xanax
c. Norflex
d. Doxidan

24. Which of the following physician's orders should you question before transcribing?

a. heparin 8,000 U sq q8h
b. Lanoxin 2.5 mg po qd
c. Nembutal 100 mg po hs prn
d. Keflin 0.5 gm q4h IV

25. The brand name for digoxin is:

a. Coumadin
b. Lasix
c. Decadron
d. Lanoxin

26. The generic name for Tagamet is:

a. Valium
b. meperidine
c. cimetidine
d. diazepam

27. Which of the following groups of drugs does *not* have an automatic stop date?

a. narcotics
b. anticonvulsants
c. antibiotics
d. anticoagulants

28. Which of the following is a screening test for tuberculosis?

a. PPD inter today
b. Cocci 1:100 now
c. Histoplasmin 0.1 ml today
d. Give IM placebo now

29. A device used by the patient to control the allowable frequency of their pain medication is a/an:

a. RX
b. PCN
c. PCA
d. CPT

30. An order for Doxidan is an order for a(an):

a. narcotic
b. antianemic
c. laxative
d. hormone

31. An order for "Compazine 10 mg IM q 6 hr N/V" is what kind of an order?

a. prn
b. standing
c. one time
d. STAT

32. An order for "Lomotil tab i qid for diarrhea" is what kind of an order?

a. prn
b. standing
c. one time
d. STAT

33. An order for Demerol 50 mg po now is what kind of an order?

a. prn
b. standing
c. one time
d. STAT

34. An order for "AquaMephyton 10 mg IM daily x 3 days" is what kind of an order?

a. prn
b. standing
c. one time
d. short order series

ANSWERS AND RATIONALE

23. (b) Xanax is a tranquilizer, a drug used to relieve anxiety without causing sleep. p. 194.

24. (b) The usual adult dose for Lanoxin is 0.125-0.25 mg. p. 199.

25. (d) The brand name for digoxin is Lanoxin. p. 197.

26. (c) The generic name for Tagamet is cimetidine. p. 196.

27. (b) Anticonvulsants do not have an automatic stop date. p. 195.

28. (a) PPD is a screening test for tuberculosis. p. 199.

29. (c) Patient controlled analgesia (PCA) is a device that allows the patient to control the administration of their pain medication. p. 178.

RX - Treatment - Prescription

PCN - Penicillin

CPT -Chest Physical Therapy

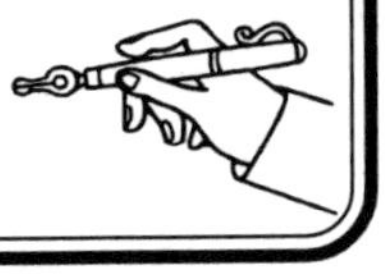

30. (c) Doxidan is a laxative. p. 198.

31. (a) PRN (whenever necessary) - the Compazine would only be given if the patient was nauseated or vomiting (N/V). pp. 142, 178, 191.

32. (a) PRN - the qualifying phrase, for diarrhea indicates that the Lomotil can be given 4 x a day (qid) if the patient has diarrhea. p. 191.

33. (d) STAT means the same as now. pp. 126, 191.

34. (d) Short order series - the AquaMephyton would be given for 3 days as directed and then discontinued. p. 191.

NOTES:

35. An order for "Lasix 40 mg IM today" would be what kind of an order?

a. prn
b. standing
c. one time
d. STAT

36. The generic name for Lasix is:

a. hydrodiuril
b. furosemide
c. chlorothiazide
d. meperidine

37. The generic name for Demerol is:

a. cimetidine
b. diazoxide
c. lidocaine
d. meperidine

38. The generic name for Tylenol is:

a. furosemide
b. diazoxide
c. acetaminophen
d. desipramine

39. An order for HCTZ is an order for a:

a. laxative
b. narcotic
c. diuretic
d. antineoplastic

40. An order for "MS" would be given to:

a. induce urination
b. relieve pain
c. reduce cholesterol formation
d. thin blood

41. To find the usual dosage or the side effects of a medication you would look in the:

a. PDR
b. Policy Manual
c. MAR
d. Medical Dictionary

42. An order is written on Monday at 0500 for "Lasix 20 mg po q 6 hr x 5 doses". When would the last dose be given if the first dose is given at 0600?

a. 6 am on Tuesday
b. 12 midnight on Monday
c. 12 noon on Monday
d. 12 noon on Tuesday

43. An order reads "Donnagel 10 cc po tid ac". The patient will receive Donnagel:

a. twice a day before meals
b. three times a day after meals
c. twice a day after meals
d. three times a day before meals

44. A medication to be administered "10 mg IM q 4 hr" should be given how many times in twenty-four hours?

a. three
b. four
c. six
d. eight

ANSWERS AND RATIONALE

35. (c) One time - the Lasix would be given as directed and then discontinued. p. 191.

36. (b) The generic name for Lasix is furosemide. p. 196.

37. (d) The generic name for Demero is meperidine. p. 193.

38. (c) The generic name for Tylenol is acetaminophen. p. 194.

39. (c) Hydrochlorothiazide (HCTZ) is a diuretic. p. 196.

40. (b) Morphine Sulfate (MS) is a narcotic and is given to relieve pain. p. 178.

41. (a) *The Physician's Desk Reference* (PDR) is where to find usual dose and side effects of medications. pp. 181, 182.

42. (a) The last dose would be given at 6 am on Tuesday (q 6 hr would be 6-12-6-12-6 for 5 doses). p. 189.

43. (d) The patient would receive the Donnagel three times a day before meals. p. 189, Table 13-1.

44. (c) The medication would be given six times in twenty-four hours (twenty-four divided by 4 equals six). p. 189, Table 13-1.

NOTES:

Chapter 14
Laboratory Orders

1. Which of the following specimens is obtained by the physician?

   a. gastric washings
   b. abdominal cavity fluid
   c. sweat
   d. wound drainage

2. The physician's order "daily Hgb" means:

   a. the test is ordered daily by the physician
   b. the test is ordered once by the physician, and requisitioned each day until discontinued
   c. the test is ordered once by the physician and done automatically by the lab until discontinued
   d. none of the above

3. The physician performs which of the following procedures to obtain a bone fluid specimen?

   a. thoracentesis
   b. lumbar puncture
   c. sternal puncture
   d. biopsy

4. An ESR is ordered from which of the following divisions within the laboratory?

   a. hematology
   b. chemistry
   c. microbiology
   d. cytology

5. Which of the following is used to determine the oxygen-carrying pigment of the blood and may be used to diagnose anemia?

   a. Hgb
   b. Hct
   c. Diff
   d. Retics

6. Which of the following is used to diagnose lupus erythematosus?

   a. APTT
   b. RBC indices
   c. Retics
   d. LE cell prep

7. Which of the following assists the physician to determine the dosage of heparin or Coumadin prescribed in anticoagulant therapy?

   a. bleeding time
   b. clotting time
   c. platelets
   d. prothrombin time

8. Which of the following tests requires the patient to be fasting?

   a. triglycerides
   b. Lytes
   c. SGOT
   d. LDH

9. You are transcribing a physician's order for electrolytes; you would order which of the following?

   a. Na, K, Cl, CO_2
   b. Na, CK, K, CO_2
   c. Na, K, Cl, Ca
   d. K, Cl, CO_2, LDH

10. Which of the following tests may be used to diagnose and/or monitor diabetes?

   a. BUN
   b. AST
   c. CPK
   d. FBS

ANSWERS AND RATIONALE

1. (b) Abdominal cavity fluid is obtained by the physician during an abdominal paracentesis. pp. 211.

2. (b) Daily Hgb means the test is ordered once by the physician and requisitioned each day until discontinued. p. 210.

3. (c) A sternal puncture, also called a bone marrow biopsy, is done by the physician to obtain bone marrow. p. 211.

4. (a) An ESR, which is a test to determine the rate at which RBC s settle out of liquid protein of the blood, is done in the hematology division within the laboratory. p. 212

5. (a) Hgb (hemoglobin) is used to determine the oxygen-carrying pigment of the blood. p. 212.

6. (d) LE cell prep is used to diagnose lupus erythematosus. p. 212.

7. (d) A prothrombin time measures the clotting ability of the blood. p. 212.

8. (a) A test for triglycerides requires the patient to be fasting. pp. 216, 218.

9. (a) Sodium (Na), potassium (K), chlorides (Cl) and carbon dioxide (CO_2) make up electrolytes. p. 217.

10. (d) FBS (fasting blood sugar) determines the amount of sugar in the blood stream after the patient has not eaten for 8 to 10 hours and is used to diagnose and/or monitor diabetes. p. 217.

NOTES:

11. You would be required to consult the patient's medication record to transcribe which of the following physician's orders?

    a. CBC and SMAC — call if K is below 3.5
    b. T & C 2 units packed cells for transfusion today
    c. Theophylline peak and trough with third dose
    d. clean catch urine for C & S

12. Which of the following are cardiac enzymes and may be ordered when a myocardial infarction is suspected?

    a. AST, CPK, LDH
    b. ALT, CPK, LDH
    c. GTT, CPK, AST
    d. AST, CPK, ALT

13. Which of the following tests is useful in diagnosing diseases that affect kidney function?

    a. Bili
    b. BUN
    c. TIBC
    d. LDH

14. You have just received the following laboratory test values by telephone. Which one should you bring to the nurse's attention immediately?

    a. WBC is 8,500
    b. K is 4.8
    c. FBS is 375
    d. PT is 14 sec.

15. For the physician's order "2 hr PP BS" it is your responsibility to:

    a. notify the lab of the time the patient last voided
    b. notify the lab when the patient has finished eating
    c. notify the nurse when the patient has finished eating
    d. none of the above

16. You would order a creatinine clearance test from which of the following laboratory divisions?

    a. serology
    b. urinalysis
    c. hematology
    d. chemistry

17. Which of the following is done to determine antibiotic treatment?

    a. Gram stain
    b. mycology studies
    c. AFB culture
    d. culture and sensitivity

18. You would order an "RA factor" from which of the following laboratory divisions?

    a. serology
    b. bacteriology
    c. hematology
    d. chemistry

19. The order "cryoprecipitates 1 unit" would be ordered from which of the following laboratory divisions?

    a. hematology
    b. chemistry
    c. bacteriology
    d. blood bank

20. Which of the following is *not* a blood bank order?

    a. packed cells, one unit
    b. give two units of platelets
    c. ASO titer
    d. normal serum albumin 5%

ANSWERS AND RATIONALE

11. (c) The medication record would need to be consulted to determine when the third dose of Theophylline will be given. The test will be ordered a half hour before and an hour after the patient receives the medication (times may vary in hospitals). p. 374.

12. (a) AST, CPK and LDH are the cardiac enzymes. p. 216.

13. (b) BUN (blood urea nitrogen) is used to diagnose diseases affecting the kidney. p. 217.

14. (c) The normal FBS value is 70 to 120, a fasting blood sugar of 375 should be brought to the nurse s attention immediately. p. 216.

15. (b) The lab must be notified when the patient has finished eating so the blood can be drawn two hours after the patient has finished eating. pp. 217, 218

> 2HR postprandial blood sugar is a test performed to determine the patient's response to carbohydrate intake. The blood specimen must be drawn two hours after the patient has finished eating.

16. (d) A creatinine clearance test is ordered from the chemistry division of the laboratory. p. 217.

17. (d) Culture and sensitivity is used to determine antibiotic treatment. p. 225.

18. (a) RA factor, a test for rheumatoid arthritis, is ordered from the serology division of the laboratory. p. 225.

19. (d) Cryoprecipitates are ordered from the blood bank within the laboratory. p. 226.

20. (c) ASO titer is a serology order. p. 226.

NOTES:

21. Which of the following orders would you communicate to the nurse to obtain?

    a. RBC indices
    b. T4
    c. UA
    d. ANA

22. Which of the following studies is used by a physician to aid in the diagnosis of diabetes?

    a. 6 HR GTT
    b. AST
    c. TIBC
    d. Creatinine clearance

23. Which of the following lab results would you report immediately to the patient's nurse?

    a. HCT is 45
    b. PT is 15 sec.
    c. FBS is 120
    d. K is 7

24. The symbol representing iron is:

    a. Ir
    b. Fi
    c. Fe
    d. In

25. Which of the following specimens would not be collected by the nurse?

    a. urine
    b. biopsies
    c. sputum
    d. wound drainage

26. Which of the following tests would require an arterial blood specimen?

    a. ASO
    b. ABG
    c. ANA
    d. APTT

27. When a patient is "fasting" the diet is:

    a. clear liq
    b. full liq
    c. water only
    d. NPO

28. Which of the following tests is a count of immature red blood cells:

    a. DIFF
    b. HGB
    c. RETICS
    d. Platelets

29. Which of the following tests is used for the diagnosis of infection.

    a. WBC
    b.. RBC
    c. HGB
    d. PLTS

30. Which of the following tests would be done to diagnose a thyroid problem?

    a. TIBC
    b. Triglycerides
    c. Uric Acid
    d. TSH

31. Which of the following lab tests would require the patient to sign a consent prior to it being ordered?

    a. FSH
    b. CEA
    c. HIV
    d. FTA

32. What procedure would be done to obtain a CSF specimen?

    a. Amniocentesis
    b. Sternal puncture
    c. Lumbar puncture
    d. Biopsy

ANSWERS AND RATIONALE

21. (c) The nurse collects the specimen for the UA (routine urinalysis). p. 227.

22. (a) 6 hr. GTT (glucose tolerance test) A test performed to determine abnormalities in glucose metabolism and is used to aid in the diagnosis of diabetes. p. 217

> For a 6 HR glucose tolerance test, the patient is in a fasting state. The test is performed over 6 hours. The patient has a FBS (fasting blood sugar) drawn to establish baseline data and then is given a large amount of glucose solution to drink. Timed blood and urine specimens are taken. At the completion of the test all urine is sent to the laboratory.

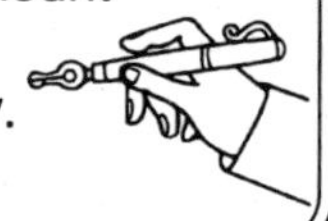

23. (d) Potassium (K) would be a critical value and should be reported immediately. Normal value is 3.5-5.0. p. 216

24. (c) Fe is the symbol for iron. p. 216.

25. (b) A biopsy specimen would be collected by a physician. p. 211.

26. (b) Arterial blood gas (ABG) would require an arterial blood specimen. pp. 255, 256.

27. (c) Fasting means the patient may have water; NPO means nothing by mouth. p. 215.

28. (c) Reticulocytes (RETICS) are the count of immature red blood cells which determines bone marrow activity. It is often used in the diagnosis of anemia. p. 215.

29. (a) White blood cells (leukocytes) (WBC) fight disease-causing organisms. p. 215.

30. (d) The thyroid-stimulating hormone (TSH) would be done to diagnose a thyroid problem. p. 218.

31. (c) Human immunodeficiency virus (HIV) is the test to detect the virus that causes AIDS (acquired immunodeficiency syndrome) and would require the patient to sign a consent prior to it being ordered. pp. 226, 115, 348, 349, 409.

32. (c) A lumbar puncture, (LP) (also called spinal tap) would be done to obtain cerebrospinal fluid (CSF). p. 211.

NOTES:

33. What lab test must be performed prior to a patient receiving a unit of packed cells?

a. T&C
b. TIBC
c. Screen
d. Complement fixation titer

34. A "Coombs test" would be ordered from which division of the lab?

a. blood bank
b. chemistry
c. microbiology
d. hematology

35. An "RPR" is a test performed to diagnose:

a. gout
b. syphilis
c. anemia
d. diabetes

36. A test performed to diagnose arthritis is a:

a. ANA
b. RA
c. CEA
d. RDW

37. A test performed to assess treatment of liver, colon or pancreatic cancer is:

a. CEA
b. ANA
c. FTA
d. complement fixation titers

38. When an order for "guaiac all stools" is written, the purpose is to detect:

a. sodium
b. fat
c. occult blood
d. sugar

39. Which of the following procedures does <u>not</u> require the patient to sign a consent?

a. lumbar puncture
b. amniocentesis
c. biopsy
d. cervical smear

40. A "CBC" would include the following tests:

a. WBC/DIFF, RBC, PT, ESR
b. WBC/DIFF, RBC, HBG, HCT
c. WBC/DIFF, PCV, ESR, APIT
d. WBC/DIFF, RBC, NA, K

41. An order for a 24 hr urine specimen would require you to order a:

a. catheter tray from SPD
b. receptacle from the lab
c. nonretention catheter from SPD
d. receptacle from SPD

42. An order for a sterile urine specimen would be obtained by the following method:

a. clean catch
b. midstream
c. catheterization
d. voided

43. Which of the following specimens should be transported to the lab immediately:

a. CSF for C&S
b. Cath UA
c. T & C 2 U PC
d. CEA

ANSWERS AND RATIONALE

33. (a) A type and crossmatch (T&C) also written as T& X match. This is a test that determines the patient's blood type and compatibility. p. 226.

34. (a) Blood bank performs the Coombs test also called DAT for direct anti globulin test. p. 226.

35. (b) Syphilis may be diagnosed by performing a rapid plasma reagin (RPR). This test is also called a VDRL (venereal disease research laboratory). p. 226.

36. (b) RA also called RA factor is a specific test for rheumatoid arthritis. p. 226.

37. (a) An elevated level of CEA (Carcinoembrynic Antigen) may indicate liver, colon, or pancreatic cancer. It is also used to assess the treatment of these conditions. p. 226.

38. (c) The purpose of an order for "guaiac all stools" is to detect occult (hidden) blood. p. 207.

39. (d) A cervical smear would not require a consent. p. 211.

40. (b) WBC (white blood cell count), RBC (red blood cell count), HGB (hemoglobin) HCT (hematocrit)/DIFF (differential) are included in a CBC. p. 212.

41. (b) An order for a 24 hr urine specimen would require you to order a receptacle from the lab. Some specimens such as a 24 hr urine specimen are kept for a period of time, therfore, a preservative is added to the collection bottle before it is sent to the unit. p. 215.

42. (c) Catheterization requires a sterile urine sample for culture and sensitivity testing. p. 227.

43. (a) CSF (cerebral spinal fluid) is obtained by an invasive procedure (lumbar puncture), therefore must be transported to the lab immediately. p. 228.

NOTES:

Chapter 15
Diagnostic Imaging Orders

1. Contrast media are used in diagnostic imaging procedures to:

   a. differentiate between bone structure
   b. clear the patient's intestinal tract
   c. increase the contrast in different body densities
   d. insure the patient does not feel any discomfort

2. The physician has ordered a BE, UGI and US of ABD. Which one should be scheduled first?

   a. UGI
   b. US of ABD
   c. BE
   d. it doesn't matter

3. A study that uses a device to record views of selected levels of the body by means of a computer and may be done with or without a contrast medium is a:

   a. thermography
   b. CT scan
   c. sialogram
   d. MUGA scan

4. A BE is a procedure performed in order to visualize the:

   a. renal pelvis
   b. small intestine
   c. upper gastrointestinal area
   d. large intestine

5. "On call" medication may be defined as medication that:

   a. is given when the patient requests it
   b. requires that the physician be called before giving
   c. requires the nurse to call the department performing the procedure on the patient for a medication order
   d. requires the nurse to give a previously ordered medication when the department performing a procedure calls the nursing station with instructions to do so

6. The physician's orders include BE, UGI and a total bone scan. Which procedure would you schedule to be done first?

   a. total bone scan
   b. BE
   c. it doesn't matter
   d. UGI

7. The procedure used to outline the kidney, renal pelvis, ureters and urinary bladder is called a(n):

   a. IVP
   b. angiogram
   c. MUGA scan
   d. UGI

8. The procedure that requires the nursing staff to administer preparation to the patient prior to the procedure is a:

   a. KUB
   b. GB study
   c. chest x-ray
   d. angiogram

ANSWERS AND RATIONALE

1. (c) Because there is little difference in density between certain organs and blood vessels, contrast media are used to increase the contrast. p. 234, 238.

2. (b) Abdominal studies using ultrasound should precede studies using barium, since barium in specific parts of the body may obscure the portion of the body being studied. p. 238.

3. (b) Computed tomography (CT) records and displays selected cross-sectional images of any body part and may be ordered with or without contrast media. p. 234, 241, 242.

4. (d) Barium enema is a procedure used to visualize the large intestine. p. 240.

5. (d) "On call" medications are prescribed by the physician to be given prior to the procedure. p. 234, 241.

6. (a) The bone scan should be done first because barium is used to perform a BE and an UGI that would obscure the view. p. 238.

7. (a) An IVP (intravenous pyelogram) outlines the kidneys, renal pelvis, ureters and urinary bladder. p. 239.

8. (b) Preparation of the patient is necessary for the GB (gallbladder study). p. 239, 240.

NOTES:

9. Which of the following scheduling of diagnostic studies is incorrect?

   a. 1. US of pelvis 2. BE 3. UGI
   b. 1. IVP 2. GB 3. BE 4. UGI
   c. 1. BE 2. UGI 3. liver and spleen scan
   d. 1. Total bone scan 2. IVP 3. BE

10. The abbreviation "PA" used with an x-ray order requires the radiographer to position the patient:

   a. either standing or lying on his/her back (supine) with the x-ray machine placed in front of the patient
   b. on his/her side
   c. lying half way onhis/her side
   d. either standing or lying on his/her stomach (prone) with the x-ray machine aimed at their back

11. An order for a L-S spine x-ray is an order for the:

   a. low-sacral area
   b. lumbo-sacral area
   c. lateral-sacral area
   d. left sacral area

12. An order written for a KUB is a request for an x-ray of the:

   a. kidneys, ureters and bladder
   b. kidneys, urethra and bladder
   c. kidneys, ureter and bile duct
   d. kidneys, uterus and bladder

13. A thermogram is:

   a. the observation of deep body structures made visible by use of a TV screen
   b. a technique that utilizes Xerox paper instead of x-ray film
   c. the image produced when the concentration of radionuclide in an organ is photographed
   d. a measurement and record of heat energy emanating from the body surface

14. Which of the following procedures requires the patient to drink sufficient water to fill the bladder prior to being sent to the diagnostic imaging department?

   a. cholecystogram
   b. retrograde pyelogram
   c. renal ultrasound
   d. IVP

15. A procedure using a powerful magnetic field and in which bones do not obscure the image as they do in x-ray is a:

   a. MRI
   b. thermogram
   c. CAT scan
   d. fluoroscopy

16. Which of the following procedures requires contrast medium?

   a. arteriogram
   b. mammogram
   c. KUB
   d. skull x-ray

17. An order of a CT scan of the L-S spine is performed in which of the following divisions of medical imaging?

   a. nuclear medicine
   b. computerized tomography
   c. endoscopy
   d. special x-ray procedures

18. A scan of the biliary tract (gallbladder) is called a:

   a. gallium scan
   b. MUGA scan
   c. cholangiogram
   d. DISIDA scan

19. Which of the following divisions of radiology would use radiopharmaceuticals (isotopes) to determine the functioning capacity of organs?

   a. magnetic resonance imaging
   b. nuclear medicine
   c. compute axial tomography
   d. ultrasound

ANSWERS AND RATIONALE

9. (c) The presence of barium would obscure visualization of the liver and spleen. Nuclear medicine studies should be done prior to barium studies for this reason. p. 238.

10. (d) PA (posterior-anterior) requires the radiographer to have the patient standing or prone with the x-ray machine aimed at the back. p. 237.

11. (b) L-S stands for lumbo-sacral. p. 234.

12. (a) KUB stands for kidneys, ureters and bladder. p. 234.

13. (d) Pathological processes such as cancer in soft tissue produce more heat than surrounding tissue. p. 234.

14. (c) The patient will be given a certain amount of water to drink and will be instructed not to void prior to a renal ultrasound. p. 242.

15. (a) MRI (magnetic resonance imaging) studies are done on selected areas of the brain, spinal cord and pelvis. A computer records cross-sectional images of the part being studied. p. 242, 243.

16. (a) An arteriogram requires an injection of contrast medium. p. 241.

17. (b) A CT scan is performed in the computerized tomography division of medical imaging. p. 241, 242.

18. (d) DISIDA scan, a nuclear medicine procedure, is a scan of the biliary tract. p. 244.

19. (b) The nuclear medicine division would use radiopharmaceuticals (isotopes). pp. 243, 244.

NOTES:

20. A lung perfusion/ventilation study is done in which of the following areas?

a. cardiology
b. pulmonary function
c. nuclear medicine
d. computerized tomography

21. Which of the following procedures requires a signed consent form by the patient?

a. mammogam
b. arthrogram
c. US of the GB
d. tomogram of the lung

22. An x-ray of the cerebral ventricles is called:

a. myelogram
b. sialogram
c. ventriculogram
d. venogram

23. A hysterosalpingogram is an x-ray of which of the following organs?

a. body tissues and salivary ducts
b. uterus and ovaries
c. ovaries and surrounding tissues
d. uterus and fallopian tubes

24. The abbreviation "LLQ" means:

a. low level quota
b. left lobe quadrant
c. left lower quadrant
d. left lumbar quadrant

25. A "routine preparation" is one that:

a. the patient routinely takes at home on a daily basis
b. is given for all x-ray procedures
c. is suggested by the radiologist to be followed to prepare the patient for a diagnostic imaging study
d. is a preparation routinely given on a particular nursing unit

26. An order for "SBFT" is:

a. special bowel follow through
b. special bladder fluoroscopy therapy
c. small bowel follow through
d. small bowel fluoroscopy transfer

27. An order for a MUGA scan would require you to send a requisition to:

a. CAT scan
b. nuclear medicine
c. MRI
d. special procedures

28. Which of the following items would not need to be noted on a radiology requisition:

a. date procedure to be done
b. mode of transportation
c. exact procedure
d. all medications ordered

29. Which of the following would be important to note on a requisition when ordering an x-ray procedure. The patient is:

a. Catholic
b. HIV Positive
c. a VIP
d. hearing impaired

30. Which of the following facts about the patient would not need to be noted on a radiology requisition:

a. may be subject to seizures
b. is taking antibiotics
c. is blind
d. is on O_2

31. A patient who has a pacemaker should not be scheduled for which of the following procedures:

a. Bone Scan
b. MRI of left humerus
c. CT of chest
d. Myelography

ANSWERS AND RATIONALE

20. (c) Lung perfusion/ventilation is a nuclear medicine study done to diagnose embolisms. p. 244.

21. (b) An arthrogram is an invasive procedure and requires a signed patient consent form. p. 241.

22. (c) A ventriculogram is an x-ray of the cerebral ventricles. p. 241.

23. (d) A hysterosalpingogram is an x-ray of the uterus and fallopian tubes. p. 241.

24. (c) LLQ means left lower quadrant. p. 234.

25. (c) "Routine preparation" is one suggested by the radiologist. p. 234.

26. (c) "SBFT" means small bowel follow through. pp. 235, 240.

27. (b) Nuclear medicine - a MUGA scan is a type of multigated angiogram cardiac scan. p. 244.

28. (d) All medications ordered - radiology would not need to know what medications the patient is taking. pp. 235, 244.

29. (d) It would be important to note that the patient is hearing impaired. p. 237.

30. (b) It would not be necessary for radiology to know that the patient was taking antibiotics. p. 237.

31. (b) MRI of left humerus. Due to the strength of the magnet and the radio frequency waves, MRI contraindications exist for patients with pacemakers, cerebral aneurysm clips or any electrically, magnetically, or mechanically activated implants. p. 242.

NOTES:

Chapter 16
Other Diagnostic Studies

1. In the order "ABG on RA" RA stands for:

   a. right arm
   b. rotating air
   c. room air
   d. right atrium

2. A vectorcardiogram is ordered from which of the following hospital departments?

   a. radiology
   b. cardiovascular diagnostics
   c. neurodiagnostics
   d. pulmonary function

3. An order for a CBG is a request for a:

   a. capillary blood gas
   b. complete blood gas
   c. cell blood gas
   d. complete blood gestation

4. Which of the following medications is to be noted when ordering an ABG?

   a. Lasix
   b. Chlor-Trimeton
   c. Coumadin
   d. Motrin

5. You would order an echocardiogram from which of the following hospital departments?

   a. radiology
   b. ultrasound
   c. pulmonary function
   d. cardiovascular diagnostics

6. An order for a "2 DM mode" refers to a(an):

   a. electrocardiogram
   b. echocardiogram
   c. vectorcardiogram
   d. x-ray view

7. The physician's order "stress test" refers to a:

   a. psychological test
   b. treadmill
   c. physical therapy exercise
   d. gastroenterology test

8. Which of the following medications is noted when ordering an EKG?

   a. Lanoxin
   b. Tigan
   c. Benadryl
   d. Tolinase

9. The physician's order for "PCG" is ordered from which of the following hospital departments?

   a. cardiovascular diagnostics
   b. pulmonary function
   c. endoscopy
   d. gastroenterology

10. The physician's order for a "Holter monitor" would be ordered from which of the following hospital departments?

    a. central service
    b. respiratory care
    c. gastroenterology
    d. cardiovascular diagnostics

11. Which of the following is an invasive procedure and therefore requires you to prepare a consent form?

    a. cardiac catheterization
    b. phonocardiogram
    c. Hollander test for vagotomy
    d. lactose tolerance test

ANSWERS AND RATIONALE

1. (c) RA stands for room air and in the order "ABG (arterial blood gases) on RA" the patient must not be on oxygen therapy. pp. 247, 255, 256.

2. (b) A vectorcardiogram is a three-dimensional study of the electrical impulses of the heart and is a cardiovascular study. p. 249.

3. (a) CBG is the abbreviation for capillary blood gas. p. 247.

4. (c) Coumadin, an anticoagulant, is noted when ordering an ABG to indicate the possibility of excessive bleeding during the puncturing of the artery to obtain the specimen. p. 255, 256.

5. (d) An echocardiogram is a cardiovascular study. p. 249.

6. (b) A 2 DM mode refers to an echocardiogram. p. 249.

7. (b) A stress test refers to a treadmill procedure. p. 249.

8. (a) Lanoxin, a cardiac medication, is noted when ordering an EKG (electrocardiogram). pp. 248, 249.

9. (a) A PCG (phonocardiogram) is ordered from the cardiovascular diagnostics department. p. 249.

10. (d) A Holter monitor is ordered from the cardiovascular department. p. 249.

11. (a) A cardiac catheterization requires an entry into the body by placing a catheter into a blood vessel and the heart and therefore is an invasive procedure. p. 250.

NOTES:

12. Doppler flow studies are ordered by the physician to determine:

   a. air flow through the lungs
   b. gastric acidity
   c. blood flow within blood vessels
   d. malabsorption of fat

13. Endoscopy is a generic term used to indicate:

   a. artificial opening into an organ
   b. visual examination of a body cavity
   c. removal of an organ
   d. visual examination of an eye

14. Which of the following procedures cannot be ordered to precede a sigmoidoscopy?

   a. EEG
   b. BE
   c. VCG
   d. SVN

15. A gastroscopy is a procedure used to:

   a. visualize the interior of the stomach
   b. measure gastric acidity
   c. create an artificial opening into the stomach
   d. visualize the intestines

16. An order for an esophageal motility and reflux study is ordered from which of the following hospital departments?

   a. respiratory care
   b. pulmonary function
   c. cardiovascular diagnostics
   d. gastroenterology

17. An order for a spirometry would be ordered from which of the following hospital departments?

   a. respiratory care
   b. pulmonary function
   c. cardiovascular diagnostics
   d. gastroenterology

18. A "BSAER" is a procedure used to record:

   a. breathing capabilities
   b. response to stimulation of a peripheral nerve
   c. hearing response
   d. involuntary eye movements

19. A "SEP" is a procedure used to record:

   a. breathing capabilities
   b. response to stimulation of a peripheral nerve
   c. hearing response
   d. involuntary eye movements

20. An order for an "ENG" would be ordered from which of the following hospital departments?

   a. endoscopy
   b. neurodiagnostics
   c. pulmonary function
   d. cardiovascular diagnostics

21. An order for "Hollander" test for vagotomy would be ordered from which of the following hospital departments?

   a. cardiovascular diagnostics
   b. pulmonary function
   c. endoscopy
   d. gastroenterology

22. A procedure done to inspect the common bile duct, biliary tract and pancreatic duct by inserting a catheter through an endoscope is called an:

   a. EGD
   b. ERCP
   c. PTHC
   d. EEG

ANSWERS AND RATIONALE

12. (c) Doppler flow studies show flow changes caused by changes within the blood vessels. p. 249.

13. (b) Endoscopy indicates the visual examination of a body cavity or hollow organ. p. 247.

14. (b) BE (barium enema) involves the filling of the colon with barium, making it impossible to visualize the interior of the sigmoid colon. p. 253.

15. (a) Gastroscopy is the visual examination of the interior of the stomach by means of a gastroscope. p. 253.

16. (d) Esophageal motility and reflux study is ordered from the gastroenterology department. p. 254.

17. (b) Pulmonary function - a spirometry is performed to measure and record the patient's lung capacity for air. p. 257.

18. (c) A BSAER (brain stem auditory evoked response) also called AER or BAER is used to record hearing response. p. 252.

19. (b) Response to stimulation of a peripheral nerve. A SEP (somatosensory evoked potentials) is performed by neurodiagnostics. p. 252.

20. (b) Neurodiagnostics - an ENG (electronystagmography) is done by placing electrodes near the patient's eyes to record involuntary eye movements. p. 252.

21. (d) Gastroenterology - a Hollander test for vagotomy is performed to determine the amount of hydrochloric acid in the patient's gastric juice after a vagotomy. p. 254.

22. (b) This procedure is called an ERCP (endoscopic retrograde cholangiopancreatography). p. 253.

EGD - esophagogastroduodenoscopy - visual inspection of the upper gastrointestinal tract is done in the endoscopy department.

PTHC - percutaneous transhepatic cholangiography - a diagnostic x-ray to visualize the biliary tract.

EEG - electroencephalogram - a recording of a patient's brain waves to study brain function is done in neurodiagnostics.

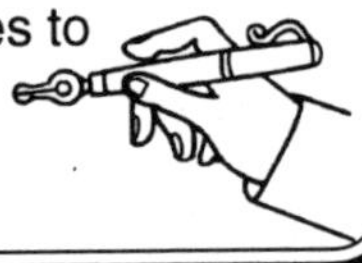

Chapter 17
Treatment Orders

1. Bryant's traction is used to treat fractures of the:

   a. humerus
   b. pelvic bone
   c. cervical vertebra
   d. femur of children three years and under

2. A type of traction used for treatment of muscle spasm is:

   a. Russell's traction
   b. cervical traction with Crutchfield tongs
   c. Bryant's traction
   d. pelvic traction, 30 lbs release PRN

3. You would order "USN 15 min qd" from which of the following hospital departments?

   a. occupational therapy
   b. central service
   c. respiratory care
   d. physical therapy

4. EMG is the abbreviation for:

   a. electromyogram
   b. ear microgram
   c. electromyelogram
   d. electromyocardiography

5. You would order "ADL" from which of the following departments?

   a. dietary
   b. physical therapy
   c. occupational therapy
   d. respiratory care

6. You would order "TENS" from which of the following hospital departments?

   a. occupational therapy
   b. physical therapy
   c. central service
   d. cardiovascular studies

7. The meaning of the abbreviation CPM is:

   a. complete patient message
   b. central pleural myogram
   c. complete posture mechanics
   d. continuous passive motion

8. Which of the following is used for hydrotherapy?

   a. diathermy
   b. range of motion
   c. aerosol
   d. whirlpool

9. You would order "ultrasound and massage to lower back" from which of the following departments?

   a. ultrasound
   b. physical therapy
   c. radiology
   d. respiratory care

10. An order for "vib and perc" is ordered from which of the following hospital departments?

    a. physical therapy
    b. rulmonary function
    c. respiratory care
    d. occupational therapy

ANSWERS AND RATIONALE

1. (d) Bryant's traction is used to treat fractured femurs of children under the age of three. p. 265.

2. (d) Pelvic traction is used for treatment of muscle spasm, sciatica, or muscle sprain. p. 265.

3. (c) USN (ultrasonic nebulizer) treatment is performed by the respiratory care department. p. 270.

4. (a) EMG is the abbreviation for electromyogram. p. 261.

5. (c) ADL (activities of daily living) is ordered from the occupational therapy department. pp. 261, 273.

6. (b) TENS (transcutaneous electrical nerve stimulation) is used to control pain and is carried out by the physical therapy department. p. 273.

7. (d) CPM is the abbreviation for continuous passive motion and is a machine used after joint replacement. pp. 261, 272.

8. (d) Whirlpool is used by physical therapy for hydrotherapy. p. 271.

9. (b) Ultrasound and massage is a heat treatment administered by the physical therapy department. p. 272.

10. (c) Vib and perc (vibration and percussion) are hand techniques used to loosen secretions within the lungs and are administered by the respiratory care department. p. 270.

NOTES:

11. An incentive spirometry would be performed by which of the following departments?

a. respiratory care
b. pulmonary function
c. occupational therapy
d. physical therapy

12. Which of the following is used in the treatment of fractures of a cervical vertebra:

a. Crutchfield's tongs
b. Steinmann's pins
c. Buck's traction
d. IPPB

13. An order for IPPB 0.5 mL Isuprel $\bar{c}$ 3 mL NS 20 cm H_2O pressure 10 min tid means:

a. respiratory care will perform treatment 10 minutes twice a day
b. physical therapy will perform treatment 10 minutes three times a day
c. physical therapy will perform treatment 10 minutes twice a day
d. respiratory care will perform treatment 10 minutes three times a day

14. In the order "SVN 0.5cc Bronkosol $\bar{c}$ 2.5cc NS 15 min qid $\bar{c}$ CPT q 4 hr", CPT means:

a. chest physical therapy
b. continuous positive treatment
c. chest positive treatment
d. compressed pressure treatment

15. The abbreviation "PEEP" included in a respiratory care order is referring to:

a. passive end expiratory position
b. promote every expiratory path
c. positive end expiratory pressure
d. prompt end expiratory press

16. An "MDI" is a:

a. monitored drug inhalation
b. metered drug inhibitor
c. metered dose inhaler
d. monitored dose inhalation

Test Taking Tip: **Sometimes the option that has the most words is correct. Item writers are aware of this and may try to avoid giving this as a clue.**

ANSWERS AND RATIONALE

11. (a) Respiratory care - incentive spirometry is a technique to encourage patients to breath deeply. p. 270.

12. (a) Crutchfield's tongs are inserted into the skull bone and a traction apparatus is applied to the tongs. p. 265.

13. (d) Respiratory care personnel will perform the IPPB (intermittent positive pressure breathing) treatment tid (3 times a day). pp. 261, 268, 143.

14. (a) Chest physical therapy is a treatment given by respiratory care personnel to loosen and remove secretions from the lung. SVN (small volume nebulizer) is a treatment similar to IPPB without positive pressure. p. 270.

15. (c) Positive end expiratory pressure (PEEP) is an order for use of a ventilator. p. 270.

16. (c) Metered dose inhaler (MDI) medication is premeasured in the pharmacy. p. 270.

NOTES:

Chapter 18
Miscellaneous Orders

1. A consultation must be requested by the:

   a. resident
   b. attending physician
   c. patient's family
   d. registered nurse

2. Information you should have available when placing a call for a consultation includes the patient's name, patient's location, person requesting the consultation, patient's diagnosis and:

   a. patient's medical record number
   b. what tests are ordered
   c. hospital name
   d. names of other doctors consulting

3. The physician may request a patient's old chart from the health record department if the patient has:

   a. previously been treated at the hospital
   b. been in the hospital a long time
   c. gone home on a pass then returned
   d. all of the above

4. In order to receive records of diagnostic studies from a patient's stay in a different hospital, a consent form must be obtained from:

   a. the previous attending physician
   b. the hospital where the records are stored
   c. the current attending physician
   d. the patient

5. A patient who is ready for discharge from the hospital but still needs nursing treatment would have his/her discharge coordinated with:

   a. VNS
   b. NWB
   c. ADL
   d. DSU

6. When scheduling a patient for a test or examination performed in a specialized hospital department or outside the hospital, it is important to indicate which of the following on the patient's kardex form?

   a. length of the test
   b. time of the test
   c. purpose of the test
   d. physician ordering the test

7. Which of the following situations would the social service department not be able to help the patient with?

   a. financial difficulties
   b. child care problems
   c. transfer to an EFC
   d. spiritual guidance

8. When arranging a temporary absence for a patient, it is necessary to:

   a. complete the discharge procedure
   b. notify social service to go to the patient's home
   c. provide transportation from the hospital
   d. cancel meals during the time of absence

ANSWERS AND RATIONALE

1. (b) A consultation must be requested by the attending physician. p. 275.

2. (c) The hospital name should be included in the information available when placing a call for consultation. p. 275.

3. (a) The old charts may be requested if the patient has been previously treated at the hospital. p. 277.

4. (d) Records of a patient's treatment in another hospital are confidential; therefore, obtaining them requires the patient's permission. p. 277.

5. (a) A patient who still needs nursing treatment after discharge would have his/her discharge coordinated with the VNS (visiting nurse service). p. 279.

6. (b) It is important to note the time of the test on the patient's kardex form. p. 279.

7. (d) Spiritual guidance is not provided by the social service department. p. 279.

8. (d) During temporary absence, all meals must be canceled. p. 280.

NOTES:

9. When the order for an in-hospital transfer of a patient has been written it is your responsibility to notify the:

   a. admitting department
   b. business office
   c. clergy
   d. central service department

10. When a patient is designated NINP, it's your responsibility to:

   a. notify the attending physician
   b. deny having the patient on the unit
   c. give status reports only about the patient
   d. none of the above

11. If asked to call the H.O. you would place the call to the:

   a. home care department
   b. resident on call
   c. attending physician
   d. patient's family

12. If a patient requests no visitors, you should notify the:

   a. physician
   b. switchboard
   c. respiratory care department
   d. visiting nurse service

13. An order for a patient to be discharged with oxygen, would require you to notify:

   a. respiratory care
   b. the patient's nurse
   c. home care department
   d. social service department

14. An order for which of the following would require the patient or legal guardian to sign a release form?

   a. temporary absence
   b. transfer to another unit
   c. transfer to another room on same unit
   d. obtain old charts from health records

Test Taking Tip: The number or letter of the correct answer may be the same as the several preceding it. When choosing your answer do not be tempted to vary your answer for this reason.

ANSWERS AND RATIONALE

9.	(a)	The admitting department must be notified of an in-hospital transfer. p. 280.
10.	(b)	NINP (no information no publication) means the unit denies having the patient. p. 282.
11.	(b)	H.O. (house officer) is the name given to the resident on call. p. 282.
12.	(b)	The switchboard must be notified if a patient requests no visitors. p. 282.
13.	(c)	An order for discharge with oxygen would require you to notify the home care department, also called discharge planning. p. 279.
14.	(a)	Temporary absence (pass to leave the hospital) would require the patient or legal guardian to sign a release. p. 280.

NOTES:

SECTION IV

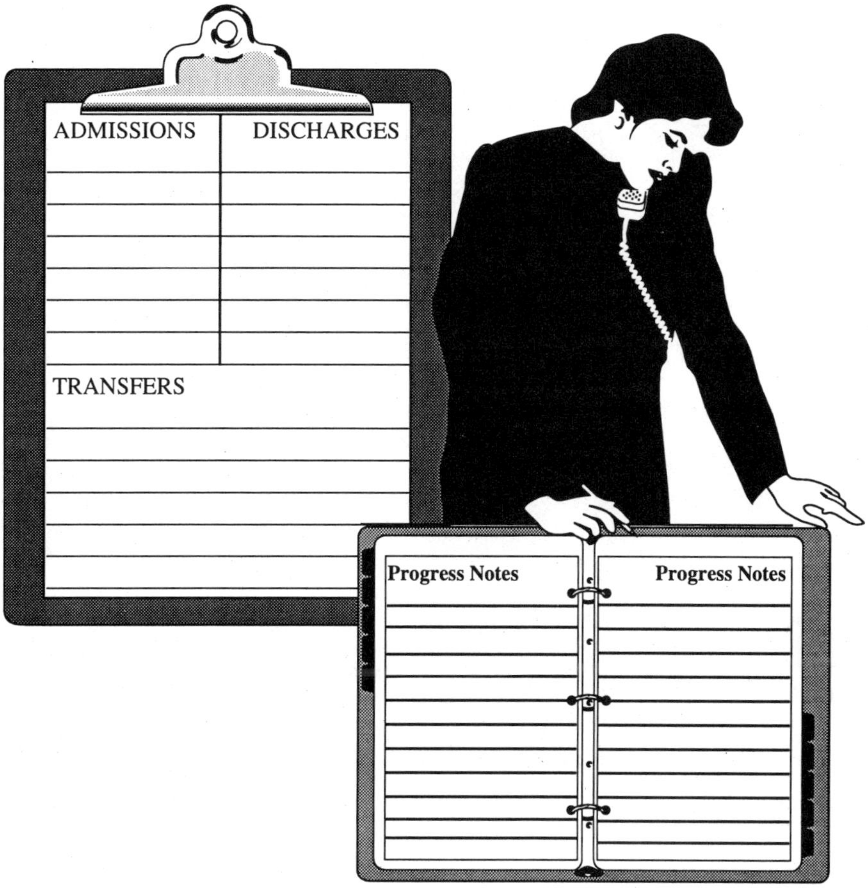

HEALTH UNIT COORDINATOR PROCEDURES

Chapter 19
Admission, Preoperative, and Postoperative Procedures

1. The admitting department is *not* responsible for which of the following when admitting the new patient?

   a. informational forms
   b. identification bracelet
   c. imprinter card or labels
   d. history and physical

2. Which of the following indicates the general services the hospital will provide?

   a. information sheet
   b. summary sheet
   c. admission agreement form
   d. progress report

3. Which of the following is *not* included on the identification bracelet?

   a. patient's name
   b. physician's name
   c. health record number
   d. patient's diagnosis

4. Which of the following is *not* a purpose of the patient's health record number?

   a. identifying chart forms
   b. billing
   c. locating previous records
   d. identifying personal belongings

5. A declaration made by the patient to family, medical staff and all concerned stating what is to be done in the event of a terminal illness is called a/an?

   a. admission agreement
   b. living will
   c. check list
   d. condition of agreement

6. A patient brought to the hospital by ambulance from an automobile accident would be admitted through the:

   a. outpatient department
   b. admitting department
   c. emergency department
   d. business office

7. The emergency department record of a patient admitted to the hospital is:

   a. placed on the patient's chart
   b. sent to the health records department
   c. filed with the emergency department records
   d. sent home with the family

8. The floor assignment for a patient whose admission is scheduled is made by the:

   a. nursing supervisor
   b. admitting department
   c. emergency department
   d. health unit coordinator

9. When the patient arrives on the nursing unit, the first thing the health unit coordinator should do is:

   a. notify the nurse
   b. call the doctor
   c. transcribe the orders
   d. call the admitting department

10. In preparing the chart for the newly admitted patient, which of the following is *not* required?

    a. imprinting the chart forms
    b. filling in the headings on the forms
    c. placing the forms behind the dividers
    d. placing the old records in the chart

ANSWERS AND RATIONALE

1. (d) The admitting department is not responsible for the history and physical. pp. 286, 287, 288.

2. (c) The form that sets forth the general services the hospital will provide is the admission agreement form. Also called C of A (conditions of admissions). pp. 286, 288.

3. (d) The patient's diagnosis is not included on the identification bracelet. p. 286.

4. (d) Personal belongings are not identified by the patient's health record number. p. 286.

5. (b) Most states now require that a patient be advised on admission to the hospital of the availability of the living will and other advance directives. pp. 285, 292.

6. (c) Admissions to the hospital as a result of a medical emergency are processed through the emergency department. p. 288.

7. (a) The emergency department record is sent to the nursing unit with the patient and placed on the patient's chart. p. 290.

8. (b) The admitting department assigns the floor and in some hospitals the bed for the scheduled admission. p. 290.

9. (a) The nurse caring for the patient should be notified first. p. 292.

10. (d) The old records do not go in the current chart. pp. 292, 277.

NOTES:

11. The health unit coordinator obtains the newly admitted patient's allergy information from the:

 a. patient him/herself
 b. conditions of admission sheet
 c. information sheet
 d. nurses' admission record

12. The anesthesiologist's preop orders would include an order for:

 a. the diet
 b. treatments
 c. enemas
 d. name of surgery

13. It is your responsibility to check that the patient's preoperative chart contains a:

 a. medication administration record
 b. progress record
 c. history and physical record
 d. vital signs record

14. A patient admitted to the hospital for observation or recovery after surgery for less than 24 hours would be admitted to which of the following units:

 a. emergency unit
 b. medical/surgical unit
 c. medical short stay unit
 d. intensive care unit

15. Upon arrival, the patient's jewelry may be placed in a valuables envelope and placed in the:

 a. hospital safe
 b. patient's bedside table
 c. unit narcotic cabinet
 d. drawer in the unit nursing station

16. The patient chart form that lists the patient's insurances and nearest relative (next of kin) is the:

 a. progress record
 b. admission agreement form
 c. information sheet
 d. summary sheet

17. A patient is admitted to your unit from the emergency department with written physician's orders. How would you find out which orders were carried out in the emergency department?

 a. call the emergency department
 b. page the doctor
 c. read the ED record
 d. ask the patient's nurse

18. Power of attorney for health care means that:

 a. the patient's attorney has the right to make medical decisions for the patient if necessary
 b. the hospital attorney will make all decisions for the patient's health care if necessary
 c. the patient's attorney will appoint someone to make health care decisions for the patient if necessary
 d. the patient has appointed another person or persons to make health care decisions for him/her if necessary

19. Same day surgery (SDS) means that the patient will:

 a. have surgery the same day that condition is diagnosed
 b. be admitted the day surgery is scheduled
 c. be discharged after surgery is completed
 d. be admitted, have surgery, and be discharged on the same day

ANSWERS AND RATIONALE

11. (d) The allergy information is obtained from the nurses' admission record. p. 292.

12. (a) Preoperative order components from the anesthesiologist are usually diet and medications. p. 296.

13. (c) It is your responsibility to check the patient's preoperative chart for the history and physical record. pp. 296, 297.

14. (c) The patient would be admitted to the medical short stay unit (MSSU). The criteria for admission to the MSSU varies from facility to facility. p. 288.

15. (a) Locked in the hospital safe. pp. 286, 289.

16. (c) The information sheet also called the face or front sheet is the form that would list the patient's insurances and nearest relative (next of kin). pp. 285, 286, 287.

17. (c) Read the emergency department (ED) record. This ED record is sent with the patient and placed in patient's chart. pp. 289, 290, 291.

18. (d) The patient has appointed another person or persons (called a proxy or agent) to make health care decisions should the patient become incapable of making decisions. p. 292.

19. (b) The patient will be admitted on the day surgery is scheduled. Also called SAD (save a day) in some hospitals. p. 295.

NOTES:

20. The surgeon has written an order for a surgery consent to read "right mastectomy". The surgery schedule lists the procedure to be done as "left mastectomy". You should:

    a. clarify the order with surgeon
    b. clarify the order with the patient
    c. prepare consent as written by surgeon and give to nurse to have signed
    d. prepare consent as listed on surgery schedule and give to nurse to have signed.

21. Which of the following if not on the patient's chart would *not* cause a patient's surgery to be delayed?

    a. signed surgery consent
    b. valuables check list
    c. history and physical record
    d. chest x-ray report

22. Which of the following forms would *not* be part of the patient surgery packet?

    a. operating room record
    b. I & O record
    c. anestesiologist's record
    d. preop check list

23. When working on a med/surg unit you receive a call from the recovery room nurse stating that a patient is returning to your unit now and will need a suction machine. You should:

    a. notify the nurse manager and order the suction machine from SPD
    b. order the suction machine from SPD stat and tell the nurse when the patient arrives
    c. notify the patient's nurse and inform him/her that a suction machine is needed
    d. notify the patient's nurse and order suction machine from SPD stat

---

Test Taking Tip: An option may be chosen on an impulse and then on review the option is changed. Avoid this. Studies have shown that the first answer that comes to mind is usually right.

ANSWERS AND RATIONALE

20. (a) Clarify the order with surgeon so any discrepancy will be corrected before the order is carried out. p. 296.

21. (b) The absence of the valuables check list would not cause a patient's surgery to be delayed. pp. 296, 297.

22. (b) The I & O (intake and output) record would not be part of the patient's surgery packet. p. 302.

23. (d) Notify the patient's nurse and order suction machine stat. p. 300.

NOTES:

Chapter 20
Discharge, Transfer, and Postmortem Procedures

1. The patient may be discharged when:

   a. the family arrives
   b. the nurses completes the discharge instructions
   c. the doctor writes the discharge order
   d. the patient states that h/she is ready to leave

2. Which of the following is *not* a procedure for a discharged patient?

   a. prepare credit slips if necessary
   b. notify dietary
   c. notify environmental services
   d. notify the attending physician

3. When preparing the discharged patient's chart for the health records department, you would *not*:

   a. check for the diagnosis on the summary sheet
   b. make sure all forms are imprinted
   c. check the nurse's discharge planning form
   d. put forms in alphabetical order

4. Transfer to an ECF differs from regular discharge in that:

   a. the admitting department must be notified
   b. additional paperwork must be done
   c. the environment services department is notified
   d. the dietary department is notified

5. Forms that go with a patient to an ECF should be:

   a. sent to the hospital clinic
   b. given to the resident
   c. sent to the physician's office to be forwarded
   d. placed in a sealed envelope and given to the ambulance driver

6. A patient leaving the hospital AMA:

   a. is leaving without physician approval
   b. has a disease of interest to the American Medical Association
   c. has asthma related allergy
   d. has appointment with medical admissions

7. When a patient is about to expire, which of the following people do *not* need to be notified?

   a. attending physician
   b. nursing supervisor
   c. family members
   d. central service department

8. An autopsy is the same as a:

   a. coroner's case
   b. postmortem
   c. death certificate
   d. none of the above

9. A hospitalized patient who dies as a result of stab wounds is considered:

   a. contaminated
   b. a coroner's case
   c. a pathologist's case
   d. a statistic

ANSWERS AND RATIONALE

1.	(c)	The patient may be discharged when the doctor writes the discharge order. p. 309..
2.	(d)	Notifying the attending physician is not necessary since s/he wrote the discharge order or gave permission for the order to be written. p. 310.
3.	(d)	It is not necessary to put the forms in alphabetical order. p. 310.
4.	(b)	A continuing care form must be filled out for a patient going to an extended care facility (ECF). pp. 310, 311, 316.
5.	(d)	Forms are placed in a sealed envelope and sent with the ambulance driver or family member to be given to the nursing staff at the extended care facility (ECF). p. 310, 311.
6.	(a)	AMA means against medical advice; therefore the patient is leaving without physician approval. pp. 311, 317.
7.	(d)	There is no need to notify the central service department. pp 311, 313.
8.	(b)	An autopsy is the same as a postmortem. pp. 311, 313.
9.	(b)	A coroner's case is one in which the patient's death is due to sudden, violent or unexplained circumstances. p. 313.

NOTES:

10. When a patient is transferred to another room in the same hospital you must:

    a. get a new health record number from admitting
    b. transcribe the transfer orders on a new kardex
    c. notify the admitting department
    d. cancel treatments and therapies

11. As the discharged patient prepares to leave the nursing unit you should:

    a. have the patient sign out
    b. obtain hospital personnel to accompany the patient
    c. routinely notify the patient's resident
    d. notify the health records department

12. In a coroner's case:

    a. family consent must be given for the autopsy
    b. consent must be obtained prior to the patient's death
    c. the doctor or coroner may obtain consent
    d. an autopsy consent is not required

13. Custodial care means that the patient:

    a. is in legal custody
    b. is taken care of by a nurse custodian
    c. requires around the clock nursing
    d. requires care of a nonmedical nature (feeding, bathing, etc.)

14. A patient appears at the nursing station and states that he is leaving the hospital without his doctor's permission. Which of the following would *not* be an appropriate response?

    a. notify the nurse manager
    b. prepare an AMA release form
    c. call transport to escort patient to the discharge area
    d. notify patient's doctor and resident

15. In transcribing a physician's order for a patient discharge you must take all of the following steps except:

    a. arranging for a follow-up appointment if the physician has requested one
    b. notifying the environmental services department the discharged patient's room should be cleaned
    c. completing the discharge summary sheet
    d. preparing the chart for health records

10. (c) You must notify the admitting department to get a new room assignment. p. 322.

11. (b) Obtain hospital personnel to accompany him/her to the discharge area. p. 310.

12. (d) An autopsy consent is not required in a coroner's case. p. 313.

13. (d) Custodial care means that the patient requires care of a nonmedical nature (feeding, bathing, etc.). p. 309.

14. (c) Call transport to escort patient to the discharge area would not be an appropriate response. p. 311.

> *An appropriate response would be to remind the patient that some medical insurances will not pay the hospitalization if the patient leaves the hospital against medical advice.*

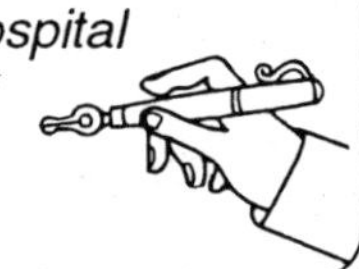

15. (c) The health unit coordinator would not complete the discharge summary sheet. p. 310.

NOTES:

Chapter 21
Routine Health Unit Coordinator Tasks

1. A physician's order for routine vital signs requires that the vital signs be checked:

   a. once a day
   b. twice a day
   c. times defined by hospital policy
   d. once a shift

2. You would record vital signs on which of the following forms?

   a. nurses' notes and activity flowsheet
   b. graphic record
   c. TPR sheet
   d. physician's progress record

3. It is important to record the vital signs in a timely manner so they are available when the:

   a. physician visits the patient
   b. next set is recorded
   c. patient is discharged
   d. patient is transferred

4. To correct a series of errors on the graphic sheet you would:

   a. cross through them and write in correct information
   b. have the nurse check the sheet
   c. notify the nurse manager
   d. recopy the graphic sheet, using the correct data

5. Which of the following is *not* a guideline for filing records in a patient's chart?

   a. separate records according to the patient's name
   b. check the name on the report with the back of the chart
   c. select the same time for filing each day
   d. call the physician's office with each report before filing

6. Records that come to the nursing unit after the patient has been discharged should be:

   a. discarded
   b. mailed to the patient
   c. given to the physician
   d. forwarded to the health records department

7. The reason daily lab tests should be ordered late in the day for the following day is:

   a. in case they are canceled
   b. so the lab won't process the order early
   c. so the nurse may change the order
   d. so the resident can check all the labs ordered

8. Daily lab tests are ordered every day until:

   a. the test results are within normal range
   b. a physician's order discontinues the lab test
   c. a nurse cancels the order
   d. the lab decides the patient no longer needs the test

ANSWERS AND RATIONALE

1. (c) Times for routine vital signs will vary according to the individual hospital policy. p. 328.

2. (b) Vital signs are recorded on the graphic sheet. pp. 328, 329.

> *Vital sign graphs are often included in the nursing record and the nurse is responsible for recording his/her patient's vital signs.*

3. (a) Recorded vital signs should be available for the physicians when they visit the patient. p. 329.

4. (d) To correct a series of errors on the graphic sheet, the entire sheet needs to be recopied using the correct data. pp. 329, 330, 332.

5. (d) It is not necessary to call the physician's office before filing each report. p. 330, 335.

6. (d) The records need to be forwarded to the health records department, where they will be added to the patient's chart. p. 335.

7. (a) Daily lab tests should be ordered late in the day for the following day in case they are canceled. p. 335.

8. (b) Daily lab tests are ordered each day until discontinued by a physician's order. p. 335.

NOTES:

9. Which of the following departments would you *not* order stock floor supplies from?

   a. central service
   b. purchasing
   c. pharmacy
   d. laboratory

10. To order a flashlight for the nursing unit, you would contact which of the following departments?:

   a. central service
   b. purchasing
   c. environmental services
   d. pharmacy

11. Alcohol sponges are obtained from which of the following departments?

   a. environmental services
   b. pharmacy
   c. central service
   d. laboratory

12. Nourishments for the nursing unit are ordered from which of the following?

   a. central service
   b. dietary
   c. environmental service
   d. cafeteria

13. The cost of linen supplies is usually absorbed by:

   a. the nursing unit budget
   b. charging for the patient's room
   c. charging of individual items to the patient
   d. none of the above

ANSWERS AND RATIONALE

9. (d) Stock floor supplies are usually not ordered from the laboratory department. pp. 335, 337.

10. (b) A flashlight is ordered from the purchasing department. pp. 337.

11. (c) Alcohol sponges are obtained from central service department. p. 337.

12. (b) Nourishments are obtained from the dietary department. p. 337.

13. (b) The cost of the linens is usually absorbed in the charge for the patient's room. p. 338.

NOTES:

Chapter 22
Other Health Unit Coordinator Tasks

1. To avoid errors in taking telephoned laboratory results, you should always:

   a. have another person listening on the line
   b. have the nurse take the results
   c. repeat the results back to the person calling
   d. have the normal values handy

2. Which of the following information is *not* usually included in the nursing unit daily census record?

   a. physician's name
   b. patient's name
   c. patient's nurse
   d. next of kin

3. An incident report is initiated if a:

   a. patient refuses a pain medication
   b. nurse is late for work
   c. medication is omitted
   d. therapy is canceled

4. Copies of incident reports are forwarded to all of the following except:

   a. quality assurance
   b. the nurse manager
   c. health records with the patient's chart
   d. risk management

5. Reverse isolation is used when a patient:

   a. has been exposed to a contagious disease
   b. has a contagious disease
   c. is susceptible to infection
   d. has a hospital-acquired infection

6. Which of the following is *not* a common hospital-acquired infection:

   a. streptococcus
   b. pseudomonas
   c. staphylococcus
   d. coccidioidomycosis

7. Disease is usually *not* spread by:

   a. air
   b. personal contact
   c. inanimate objects
   d. body excretion

8. When a patient suffers a code arrest it means:

   a. his/her heart or breathing has stopped
   b. his/her insurance has been canceled
   c. s/he are under arrest
   d. none of the above

9. When a patient suffers a code arrest, you should first call the:

   a. attending physician
   b. resident
   c. nursing supervisor
   d. switchboard operator

10. When a patient suffers a code arrest, your main responsibility is to:

    a. stay at the desk
    b. perform CPR
    c. call each department to send someone to the floor
    d. go to ICU and arrange for a bed

ANSWERS AND RATIONALE

1. (c) To avoid errors, always read the laboratory values you have recorded back to the person in the laboratory. pp. 341, 343.

2. (d) Next of kin is not usually included in the daily nursing unit census record. pp. 343, 344.

3. (c) Incident reports are required for accidents, thefts, errors of omission or errors in administration of patient medication or treatments. p. 343.

4. (c) Copies of the incident report would be forwarded to all except for the health records with the patient's chart. Incident reports are never a part of the patient's permanent record. p. 343.

5. (c) Reverse isolation is a precautionary measure that is practiced in order to prevent a patient with impaired or low resistance to disease from being infected. p. 346.

> *Reverse isolation may also be called protective isolation.*

6. (d) The three organisms usually responsible for hospital-acquired infections are streptococcus, staphylococcus and pseudomonas. p. 346.

7. (c) Disease may be spread by air, personal contact and body excretions. p. 346.

8. (a) A code arrest means that the patient's heart or breathing has stopped. p. 349.

9. (d) The switchboard operator is notified immediately to announce the code. The code team will respond to the code when it is announced by the operator. p. 349.

10. (a) Your responsibilities during a code arrest are performed from the desk area. (Your responsibilities include directing the code team to the room, ordering tests and procedures and placing necessary phone calls). p. 349.

NOTES:

11. In the event of a hospital fire the staff is:

   a. notified by code name and/or number
   b. notified by a fireman
   c. not notified
   d. none of the above

12. An example of a situation where a hospital would institute a disaster procedure is:

   a. 20% of the staff calling in sick
   b. a train wreck
   c. a car accident with two injuries
   d. a trauma patient brought in by helicopter

13. All of the following procedures are included in universal precautions except:

   a. gowns and masks are worn when caring for all patients.
   b. gloves are worn by health care workers when drawing blood from a patient.
   c. patient specimens are bagged and labeled before given to the HUC
   d. goggles are worn by health care workers if splashing of blood or body fluids is expected

14. AIDS stands for:

   a. acquired immunodeficiency syndrome
   b. activated immuno virus disease symptoms
   c. activated immmunodeficiency syndrome
   d. acquired immuno disease syndrome

15. Which of the following diagnosis may *not* be entered on the computer or on requisitions?

   a. Hepatitis
   b. AIDS
   c. Alzheimer's
   d. PID

16. A patient would be placed in AFB isolation to prevent transmission of:

   a. AIDS
   b. RSV
   c. TB
   d. HBV

17. A condition also spread by body fluids that is more contagious than AIDS is:

   a. HBV
   b. RA Factor
   c. PID
   d. URI

18. A laboratory phlebotomist informed you that h/she performed a lab test on the wrong patient. After notifying the appropriate nurses and doctors, you would:

   a. call the lab supervisor
   b. call risk management
   c. prepare an incident report
   d. notify the involved patient's families.

ANSWERS AND RATIONALE

11. (a) A code name and/or number is used to avoid using the term "fire." p. 350.

12. (b) Disasters may occur during a flood, fire, bombing or an accident such as a train or plane wreck. p. 350.

13. (a) Gowns and masks are not required for all patients and are used only if necessary. p. 348.

14. (a) AIDS stands for: acquired immunodeficiency syndrome. p. 348.

15. (b) AIDS (acquired immunodeficiency syndrome) would not be entered on the computer or on requisitions. pp. 348, 349.

> *Laws regarding AIDS and confidentiality vary from state to state, as do laws regarding disclosure of HIV-positive persons. When in doubt, do not disclose information. In most health care facilities, guidelines such as not entering the AIDS diagnosis on the computer, have been established to assist the health care worker.*

16. (c) A patient would be placed in isolation to prevent transmission of TB (tuberculosis). AFB stands for acid-fast bacilli which cause tuberculosis. pp. 347, 225.

> *AIDS - acquired immunodeficiency syndrome*
> *RSV - respiratory syncytial virus*
> *HBV - hepatitis B virus*

17. (a) HBV (hepatitis B virus) is also spread by body fluids and is more contagious than AIDS. pp. 226, 348.

> *RA Factor - a laboratory test to diagnose rheumatoid arthritis*
> *PID - pelvic inflammatory disease*
> *URI - upper respiratory infection*

18. (c) Documentation of all incidents is important in the case of a lawsuit arising from them. Incidents are trended and studied in an attempt to prevent similar incidents from happening in the future. pp. 343, 345, 346.

SECTION V

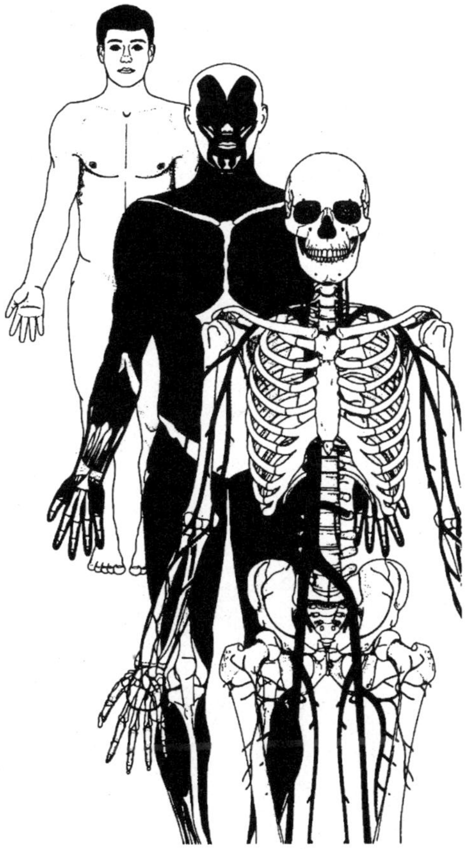

INTRODUCTION TO ANATOMIC STRUCTURES, MEDICAL TERMS, AND ILLNESS

Chapter 23
Medical Terminology, Basic Human Structure, Diseases, and Disorders (Continued)

UNIT II: Body Structure and Skin

1. The basic unit of all life is the:

   a. cell
   b. cytoplasm
   c. heart
   d. skin

2. The three main parts of a cell are:

   a. tissue, cytoplasm, cell membrane
   b. tissue, organ, system
   c. protoplasm, cell membrane, nucleus
   d. cell membrane, cytoplasm, nucleus

3. Tissue is made up of:

   a. similar cells
   b. different cells
   c. similar organs
   d. different organs

4. Which of the following is a body organ?

   a. cell
   b. tissue
   c. ureter
   d. nucleus

5. The spleen is located in which of the following cavities?

   a. cranial
   b. thoracic
   c. abdominal
   d. pelvic

6. The directional term for "in front of" is:

   a. posterior
   b. anterior
   c. cranial
   d. lateral

7. The term "caudal" means:

   a. below
   b. above
   c. in front of
   d. in back of

8. The term which means "pertaining to the side" is:

   a. lateral
   b. medial
   c. anterior
   d. posterior

9. Which of the following is *not* a function of the skin?

   a. protection from pathogenic microorganisms
   b. regulation of body temperature
   c. passage of sensory messages
   d. exchange of gases

10. The outer layer of the skin is called:

    a. epidermis
    b. dermis
    c. subcutaneous
    d. porous

ANSWERS AND RATIONALE

1. (a) The basic unit of all life is the cell. p. 358.

2. (d) The three main parts of a cell are the cell membrane, cytoplasm and nucleus. p. 358.

3. (a) Tissue is made up of similar cells. pp. 358, 359.

4. (c) Ureter, a tube which leads from each kidney to the bladder, is a body organ. pp. 359, 443.

5. (c) The spleen is located in the abdominal cavity. pp. 359, 408.

6. (b) Anterior means in front of (or ventral). p. 360.

7. (a) Caudal means below (or inferior). p. 360.

8. (a) Lateral means pertaining to the side. p. 360.

9. (d) Exchange of gases is a function of the respiratory system. p. 360.

10. (a) The epidermis, which contains no blood vessels, is the outer layer of the skin. The dermis is often referred to as the true skin. p. 360.

NOTES:

11. Which of the following is the death of body tissue caused by a lack of blood supply to an area of the body?

a. abscess
b. cancer
c. gangrene
d. laceration

12. The term which means "disease producing" is:

a. pathology
b. carcinogenic
c. pathogenic
d. carcinoma

13. The term which means "resembling hair" is:

a. cytoid
b. trichoid
c. dermatoid
d. sternoid

14. A tumor composed of connective tissue is called:

a. lipoma
b. sarcoma
c. myoma
d. epithelioma

15. The term which means "study of cells" is:

a. dermatology
b. histology
c. cytology
d. pathology

16. To refer to internal organs, you would use the term:

a. epithelial
b. visceral
c. dermal
d. abdominal

Test Taking Tip: **An option may be chosen on an impulse and then on review the option is changed. Avoid this. Studies have shown that the first answer that comes to mind is usually right.**

ANSWERS AND RATIONALE

11. (c) Gangrene is the death of body tissue caused by a lack of blood supply to an area of the body. p. 363.

12. (c) Pathogenic means disease producing. p. 366.

13. (b) Trichoid means resembling hair. p. 366.

14. (b) Sarcoma is a tumor composed of connective tissue. p. 367.

15. (c) Cytology means study of cells. p. 366.

16. (b) Visceral means internal organs. p. 367.

NOTES:

Chapter 23
Medical Terminology, Basic Human Structure, Diseases, and Disorders (Continued)

UNIT III: The Musculoskeletal System

17. The patient was admitted to the hospital with a "fractured upper jaw" or:

    a. maxilla
    b. mandible
    c. malleus
    d. metacarpal

18. The pelvic bones are composed of which of the following?

    a. lumbar, sacrum, coccyx
    b. ilium, ischium, pubis
    c. ischium, ilium, sacrum
    d. pubis, ischium, ileum

19. Which of the following bones form the upper sides of the cranium?

    a. temporal
    b. ethmoid
    c. sphenoid
    d. parietal

20. The first seven vertebrae which form the neck are:

    a. cervical
    b. thoracic
    c. lumbar
    d. clavicle

21. The bones which form the wrist are:

    a. tarsals
    b. metatarsals
    c. carpals
    d. metacarpals

22. The lower arm bone, thumb side is the:

    a. ulna
    b. humerus
    c. radius
    d. tibia

23. Muscles are attached to bone by:

    a. ligaments
    b. tendons
    c. nerves
    d. joints

24. Which of the following may be performed for treatment of a "herniated nucleus pulposus"?

    a. arthroplasty
    b. laminectomy
    c. laparotomy
    d. chondrectomy

25. A fracture with a broken bone and an open wound in the skin is called:

    a. simple
    b. compound
    c. greenstick
    d. closed

26. Tough bands of tissue that connect one bone to another bone at a joint are called:

    a. periosteum
    b. ligament
    c. tendon
    d. muscle

ANSWERS AND RATIONALE

17. (a) Maxilla is the name for upper jaw bone. p. 369.

18. (b) The pelvic bones are composed of the ilium, ischium and pubis. p. 372. The ileum is a portion of the small intestine. p. 421.

19. (d) The parietal bones form the upper sides of the cranium. pp. 369, 370.

20. (a) The cervical vertebrae form the neck. p. 369, 370

21. (c) The carpals form the wrist. p. 371.

22. (c) The radius is the lower arm bone, thumb side. p. 371.

23. (b) Muscles are attached to bone by tendons. p. 372.

24. (b) A laminectomy, which is the surgical removal of a portion of the vertebra, may be performed as a treatment for herniated nucleus pulposus, also called a herniated or slipped disc. p. 373.

25. (b) Open or compound is a fracture with a broken bone and an open wound. p. 373.

26. (b) Ligaments connect bones at a joint. p. 372.

NOTES:

27. The term which means "pertaining to the thigh bone" is:

    a. tibial
    b. humeral
    c. femoral
    d. femeral

28. The term which means "pertaining to below the ribs" is:

    a. subscapular
    b. suprascapular
    c. subcostal
    d. sublingual

29. Which of the following terms means "surgical incision into the collar bone"?

    a. chondrectomy
    b. costectomy
    c. craniotomy
    d. clavicotomy

30. The progressive crippling disease of the muscle is:

    a. muscular dystrophy
    b. muscular atrophy
    c. myocardial infarction
    d. multiple sclerosis

31. Which of the following terms means "pertaining to between the vertebrae"?

    a. intravertebral
    b. vertebrocostal
    c. vertebrectomy
    d. intervertebral

32. The instrument used to visualize a joint is:

    a. arthrogram
    b. arthroscope
    c. arthroscopy
    d. arthrotomy

33. The physician would perform which of the following to obtain bone marrow for study?

    a. sternoclavicular
    b. sternocostal
    c. sternal puncture
    d. sternotomy

34. The "process of recording electric potential of muscle activity" is:

    a. electromyograph
    b. electromyography
    c. electromyogram
    d. none of the above

35. The term which means "inflammation of the cartilage" is:

    a. chondritis
    b. arthritis
    c. arthrosis
    d. chondrogenic

ANSWERS AND RATIONALE

27. (c) Femoral means pertaining to the thigh bone. pp. 376,377.

28. (c) Subcostal means pertaining to below the ribs. p. 379.

29. (d) Clavicotomy means surgical incision into the collar bone. p. 379.

30. (a) Muscular dystrophy is a crippling disease of the muscle. p. 379.

31. (d) Intervertebral means pertaining to between the vertebrae. *Inter* means between, whereas *intra* means within. p. 379.

32. (b) Arthroscope is the instrument used to visualize a joint. *Scope* means instrument, whereas *"scopy"* means the examination. p. 380.

33. (c) Sternal puncture is performed to obtain bone marrow. p. 380.

34. (b) Electromyography is the process of recording electric potential of muscle activity. p. 380.

35. (a) Chondritis means inflammation of the cartilage. p. 379.

NOTES:

Chapter 23
Medical Terminology, Basic Human Structure, Diseases, and Disorders (Continued)

UNIT IV: The Nervous System

36. The brain is divided into three main parts, consisting of the:

    a. cerebrum, spinal cord, brain stem
    b. cerebrum, cerebellum, brain stem
    c. brain stem, nerves, cerebellum
    d. cerebrosis, cerebellum, brain stem

37. Which of the following transmits nerve impulses from the brain to the spinal cord?

    a. ventricles
    b. dura mater
    c. sensory neurons
    d. motor neurons

38. The ventricles produce which of the following?

    a. nerve impulses
    b. red blood cells
    c. cerebrospinal fluid
    d. electrical stimuli

39. Following a CVA, the patient is experiencing loss of memory and motor function. This is probably caused by tissue damage to the:

    a. cerebellum
    b. cerebrum
    c. brain stem
    d. spinal cord

40. The spinal cord extends from the brain to:

    a. between the first and second lumbar vertebrae
    b. below the fourth lumbar vertebra
    c. the sacrum
    d. between the tenth and eleventh thoracic vertebrae

41. Injury to the spinal cord may result in loss of:

    a. vision
    b. hearing
    c. memory
    d. muscle function

42. The meninges are made up of which of the following layers?

    a. dura mater, arachnoid, pia mater
    b. dura mater, ventricles, pia mater
    c. dura mater, spinal cord, pia mater
    d. dura mater, subarachnoid space, pia mater

43. A patient who complains of loss of balance may have a disease or condition of the:

    a. brain stem
    b. cerebellum
    c. cerebrum
    d. aqueous humor

ANSWERS AND RATIONALE

36. (b) The brain consists of the cerebrum, cerebellum and brain stem. p. 387.

37. (d) Motor neurons carry impulses away from the brain, whereas the sensory neurons transmit impulses to the brain. p. 387.

38. (c) The ventricles produce cerebrospinal fluid, which surrounds the brain and spinal cord and acts as a cushion. p. 387.

39. (b) The cerebrum contains sensory, motor, sight and hearing centers. Memory, intellect, judgment and emotional reactions also take place in the cerebrum. p. 387.

40. (a) The spinal cord extends to between the first and second lumbar vertebrae. p. 387.

41. (d) Injury to the spinal cord may interfere with the transmitting of motor impulses, resulting in loss of muscle function. p. 387.

42. (a) Dura mater, arachnoid and pia mater make up the meninges. p. 387.

43. (b) Balance is a function of the cerebellum. p. 387.

NOTES:

44. Impaired blood supply to parts of the brain is called a stroke or:

a. cerebral palsy
b. coronary vascular accident
c. coronary thrombosis
d. cerebrovascular accident

45. Which of the following is considered a warning sign for stroke and is characterized by recurrent episodes of decreased neurological function?

a. CVA
b. CHF
c. T I A
d. TUR

46. Which of the following is characterized by loss of memory, restlessness and inability to carry out purposeful movement?

a. Parkinson's disease
b. Alzheimer's disease
c. Cushing's disease
d. Addison's disease

47. Following a spinal cord injury the patient had paralysis of her legs or:

a. paraplegia
b. quadriplegia
c. hemiplegia
d. none of the above

48. Select the correct spelling of the following medical term.

a. neurorrhaphy
b. neurorrhapy
c. neurorraphy
d. neurorhaphy

49. A patient diagnosed as having "multiple sclerosis" would seek treatment from a:

a. urologist
b. orthopedist
c. neurologist
d. psychiatrist

50. A viral disease which attacks the gray matter of the spinal cord is:

a. poliomyelitis
b. epilepsy
c. encephalitis
d. cerebellitis

51. Which of the following would be printed on a surgical schedule?

a. neuroma
b. neuritis
c. neuralgia
d. neuroplasty

52. The medical term for "inflammation of the brain" is:

a. encephalitis
b. meningitis
c. poliomyelitis
d. cerebellitis

53. Which of the following conditions involve the herniation of the spinal cord and meninges?

a. encephalocele
b. meningomyelocele
c. cerebral palsy
d. meningomyelorrhea

54. A procedure that may be done to determine brain death is:

a. electroencephalogram
b. pneumoencephalogram
c. echoencephalogram
d. none of the above

ANSWERS AND RATIONALE

44. (d) Cerebrovascular accident (CVA) is a result of impaired blood supply to parts of the brain. p. 387.

45. (c) TIA or (transient ischemic attack) is characterized by double vision, slurred speech, weakness in the legs and dizziness, lasting from seconds to 24 hours and then clearing. p. 387.

46. (b) Symptoms of Alzheimer's disease, which usually begins in mid-life and is progressive, include memory loss, restlessness and inability to carry out purposeful movement. p. 388.

47. (a) Paraplegia is the paralysis of the legs and sometimes the lower part of the body and is usually the result of a spinal cord injury. p. 391.

48. (a) Neurorrhaphy is the correct spelling. Note that the suffix orrhaphy, which means to suture, has two r's and two h's. p. 391.

49. (c) A patient with multiple sclerosis, a degenerative disease involving the brain and spinal cord, would seek treatment from a neurologist, one who treats diseases of the nervous system. p. 391.

50. (a) Poliomyelitis is a viral disease that attacks the gray matter of the spinal cord. p. 391.

51. (d) Neuroplasty is a surgical term; therefore it would appear on the surgery schedule. p. 391.

52. (a) Encephalitis means inflammation of the brain. Cerebellitis means inflammation of the cerebellum only and not the whole brain. p. 391.

53. (b) Meningomyelocele means herniation of the spinal cord and meninges. p. 391.

54. (a) Electroencephalogram (EEG) is a tracing or recording of the electric impulses of the brain. p. 392.

NOTES:

55. The procedure used to obtain a cervical smear is a:

a. pelvic examination
b. lumbar puncture
c. myringotomy
d. abdominocentesis

56. One who studies the mind is a:

a. neurologist
b. psychologist
c. psychiatrist
d. physiatrist

57. Which of the following refers to a mental disorder?

a. neurosis
b. psychosis
c. psychosomatic
d. neurotic

58. A condition recognized by symptoms including muscle rigidity, tremors, and a shifting gait is:

a. Alzheimer's disease
b. Parkinson's disease
c. Graves' disease
d. Diabetes Mellitus

Test Taking Tip: Do not spend more than a minute or two on a question. If you are having difficulty selecting an answer, note that you did not answer the question, move on to the next, and then return to the unanswered questions when you have completed the exam. Subsequent questions may give you a clue to the correct answer.

ANSWERS AND RATIONALE

55. (a) Pelvic examination is used to obtain a cervical smear. Also called pap test. p. 211.

56. (b) A psychologist is one who studies the mind, whereas a psychiatrist is a physician who deals with the study, treatment and prevention of mental illness. p. 395.

57. (b) Psychosis is a mental disorder. p. 395.

58. (b) Parkinson's disease, also called Shaking Palsy, is one of the most crippling diseases in the United States. p. 388.

Alzheimer's Disease is characterized by confusion, loss of memory, restlessness, hallucinations and the inability to carry out purposeful movement.

Graves' Disease is a form of hyperthyroidism.

Diabetes Mellitus is a disease that results in the inability of the body to store and use carbohydrates in the usual manner.

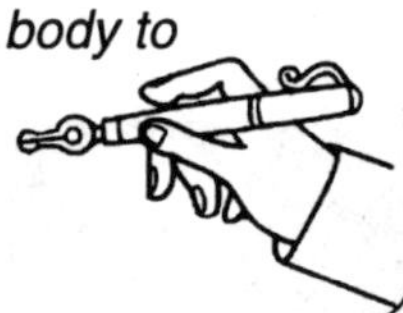

NOTES:

Chapter 23
Medical Terminology, Basic Human Structure, Diseases, and Disorders (Continued)

UNIT V: The Eye and the Ear

60. The transparent membrane that lines the upper and lower eyelid and the anterior portion of the eye is called:

   a. choroid
   b. conjunctiva
   c. sclera
   d. cornea

61. The middle layer of the eye is called the:

   a. choroid
   b. retina
   c. sclera
   d. cornea

62. The anterior middle portion of the choroid is made up of the:

   a. sclera and cornea
   b. pupil and ciliary muscle
   c. iris and pupil
   d. iris and ciliary muscle

63. The cornea is known as the:

   a. white of the eye
   b. transparent part of the sclera
   c. regulator of the shape of the eye
   d. protector of the eye from harmful bacteria

64. The dilation and contraction of the pupil of the eye are regulated by the muscles of the:

   a. iris
   b. pupil
   c. choroid
   d. sclera

65. The eye receives light rays that are focused on the:

   a. choroid
   b. cornea
   c. lens
   d. retina

66. The large posterior space behind the lens is filled with a jelly-like substance called:

   a. aqueous humor
   b. vitreous humor
   c. lens
   d. ciliary body

67. Which of the following is *not* in the pathway of light?

   a. pupil
   b. lens
   c. iris
   d. vitreous humor

68. Phacoemulsification is a surgical procedure used to treat:

   a. glaucoma
   b. strabismus
   c. retinal detachment
   d. cataracts

69. Maintaining equilibrium is a function of the:

   a. cerebrum
   b. brain stem
   c. ear
   d. thymus gland

ANSWERS AND RATIONALE

60. (b) The conjunctiva lines the eye and serves to protect it from harmful bacteria. p. 397.

61. (a) The middle layer of the eye is the choroid, which contains blood vessels that supply nutrients to the eye. p. 397.

62. (d) The iris and ciliary muscle make up the anterior middle portion of the choroid. The iris is the colored portion, which regulates light entering the eye. p. 397.

63. (b) The cornea is the transparent part of the sclera which lies over the iris and allows light rays to enter. p. 397.

64. (a) The iris, the colored portion of the eye, regulates the dilation and contraction of the pupil. p. 397.

65. (d) The light rays received by the eye are focused on the retina. p. 397.

66. (b) The substance that fills the large posterior space behind the lens is called vitreous humor. Its function is to maintain the shape of the eyeball and to assist in bending light rays. p. 397.

67. (c) The iris is not in the pathway of light. p. 397.

68. (d) Phacoemulsification, the use of ultrasonic vibrations to break the lens into pieces which are then aspirated, is used to treat cataracts. p. 397.

69. (c) Maintaining equilibrium and hearing are the two functions of the ear. p. 397.

NOTES:

70. The small shaped structure next to the oval window in the inner ear is the:

a. semicircular canals
b. cochlea
c. auditory nerve
d. incus

71. The eustachian tube leads from the pharynx to the:

a. middle ear
b. outer ear
c. inner ear
d. none of the above

72. The ossicles consist of the:

a. malleus, incus and stapes
b. malleus, stapes and cochlea
c. incus, stapes and cochlea
d. incus, stapes and tympanic membrane

73. Blepharoplasty is the surgical repair of the:

a. lip
b. eyelid
c. iris
d. eyebrow

74. The word root for cornea is:

a. irid/o
b. kerat/o
c. retin/o
d. blephar/o

75. Surgery for removal of a clouded lens is:

a. ophthalmectomy
b. cataract extraction
c. enucleation
d. sclerotomy

76. Which of the following is the result of a weakness in the eye muscle?

a. glaucoma
b. strabismus
c. retinal detachment
d. keratocele

77. The correct spelling of the term which means "discharge from the ear" is:

a. otorrhea
b. otorhea
c. otorrea
d. otarrhea

78. Which of the following instruments is kept on the nursing unit?

a. proctoscope
b. bronchoscope
c. ophthalmoscope
d. arthroscope

79. A child suffering from "otitis media" would complain of pain in the:

a. ear
b. nose
c. throat
d. eye

80. The medical term for "pinkeye" is:

a. conjunctivitis
b. otitis media
c. sclerokeratitis
d. scleritis

81. A middle ear infection is causing pressure on the eardrum. An incision into the eardrum to release the pressure and to allow for drainage is called:

a. blepharotomy
b. sclerotomy
c. myringotomy
d. stapedectomy

ANSWERS AND RATIONALE

70. (b) The cochlea, shaped like a snail, is the structure next to the oval window in the ear. p. 398.

71. (a) The eustachian tube, which leads from the middle ear to the pharynx, equalizes pressure on both sides of the tympanic membrane. p. 398.

72. (a) The ossicles are made up of the malleus, incus and stapes. p. 398.

73. (b) Blepharoplasty is the surgical repair of the eyelid. p. 401.

74. (b) The word root for cornea is kerat/o. p. 400.

75. (b) Cataract extraction is surgery to remove a clouded lens. p. 397.

76. (b) Strabismus or crossed eyes is a condition resulting from weakness of the eye muscle. p. 402.

77. (a) Otorrhea is the correct spelling. Orrhea is from the grouping of "orrh" suffixes which also includes orrhagia and orrhaphy. p. 401.

78. (c) The ophthalmoscope is kept on the nursing unit. The other instruments listed are used for more complex examination and therefore are stored in special examining rooms. p. 402.

79. (a) Otitis media is the inflammation of the middle ear; therefore the child would experience pain in the middle ear. p. 402.

80. (a) Conjunctivitis is the medical term for pinkeye. p. 402.

81. (c) Myringotomy means incision into the tympanic membrane or eardrum. p. 401.

NOTES:

Chapter 23
Medical Terminology, Basic Human Structure, Diseases, and Disorders (Continued)

UNIT VI: The Circulatory System

82. The partition dividing the heart into the right and left sides is called the:

    a. septum
    b. bicuspid valve
    c. tricuspid valve
    d. mitral valve

83. Which of the following body systems is responsible for carrying food, oxygen, waste and other materials needed for cell function?

    a. digestive
    b. circulatory
    c. endocrine
    d. respiratory

84. Which of the following carries oxygenated blood?

    a. inferior vena cava
    b. aorta
    c. superior vena cava
    d. pulmonary artery

85. Blood returns to the right atrium of the heart through which of the following?

    a. aorta
    b. pulmonary vein
    c. superior vena cava
    d. pulmonary artery

86. The exchange of substances between the blood and body cells takes place while the blood is in the:

    a. venules
    b. arterioles
    c. lungs
    d. capillaries

87. The fluid portion of the blood is called:

    a. platelets
    b. plasma
    c. leukocytes
    d. erythrocytes

88. A sternal puncture is performed by physicians to determine:

    a. bone density
    b. erythrocyte production
    c. bone marrow capacity
    d. leukocyte production

89. To diagnose appendicitis, the doctor may order which of the following laboratory tests to determine the presence of infection in the body?

    a. white blood cell count
    b. red blood cell count
    c. platelet count
    d. hemoglobin

90. The prime function of platelets is to:

    a. aid in clotting blood
    b. carry oxygen
    c. fight pathogenic microorganisms
    d. none of the above

91. Which of the following pumps blood through the pulmonary artery?

    a. right atrium
    b. left ventricle
    c. right ventricle
    d. left atrium

82. (a) The septum divides the heart into the right and left sides. p. 405.

83. (b) The circulatory system. The heart pumps the blood, which carries food, oxygen, waste and other materials through the blood vessels to the lungs and other body cells. pp. 405, 408.

84. (b) The aorta, the largest artery in the body, carries oxygenated blood away from the left ventricle of the heart. pp. 405, 408.

85. (c) The superior and inferior venae cavae are large veins through which the blood returns to the atrium from the body. pp. 405, 408.

86. (d) While the blood is in the capillaries, microscopic thin-walled blood vessels, the exchange of nutrients, oxygen and carbon dioxide between the blood and body cells takes place. p. 405.

87. (b) Plasma is the fluid portion of the blood. It is approximately 90% water. Blood cells are suspended in the plasma. p. 407.

88. (b) Erythrocytes are produced by the red bone marrow found in the flat bones of the body such as the sternum. A sternal puncture is performed to obtain a red bone marrow specimen in order study its ability to produce erythrocytes. pp. 407, 408.

89. (a) White blood cells or leukocytes fight against disease-causing bacteria. An elevated white blood count may indicate infection in the body. p. 408.

90. (a) The prime function of platelets is to aid in clotting the blood. p. 408.

91. (c) The right ventricle pumps blood through the pulmonary arteries, whereas the left ventricle pumps blood through the aorta to the body parts. p. 408.

NOTES:

92. The bicuspid valve is located between the:

a. left atrium and left ventricle
b. right atrium and right ventricle
c. right ventricle and pulmonary artery
d. left ventricle and aorta

93. As the blood is circulating through the heart, it travels from the pulmonary vein to the:

a. right atrium
b. left ventricle
c. right ventricle
d. left atrium

94. A function of the spleen is to:

a. store blood for emergency use
b. produce platelets
c. produce insulin
d. none of the above

95. Buildup of plaque on the arterial walls which leads to blockage is called:

a. arteriosclerosis
b. aneurysm
c. atherosclerosis
d. arteriostenosis

96. The patient is scheduled for the surgical removal of enlarged veins in the rectal area or:

a. herniorrhaphy
b. hemorrhoidectomy
c. splenectomy
d. angiorrhaphy

97. Which of the following is commonly referred to as a heart attack?

a. coronary thrombosis
b. pulmonary thrombosis
c. coronary aneurysm
d. myocardial infarction

98. A disease characterized by rapid abnormal production of white blood cells is:

a. hemophilia
b. anemia
c. splenomegaly
d. leukemia

99. The medical term for excision of the spleen is:

a. spleenectomy
b. spleenopexy
c. splenectomy
d. splenopexy

100. Which of the following is the medical term for inflammation of a vein as a result of a clot?

a.. thrombosis
b. arteriothrombosis
c. thrombophlebitis
d. embolism

101. A cardiologist would treat which of the following conditions?

a. hypertension
b. uremia
c. stomatitis
d. hepatoma

102. The physician ordered an x-ray of blood vessels with dye used as contrast medium or a(n):

a. angiogram
b. aortogram
c. arteriogram
d. venogram

103. The process of recording electrical impulses of the heart is:

a. electrocardiograph
b. electrocardiography
c. electrocardiogram
d. none of the above

104. A disease that attacks the immune system of patients, making them very susceptible to infection is:

a. CAD
b. Anemia
c. CHF
d. AIDS

ANSWERS AND RATIONALE

92. (a) The bicuspid valve separates the left atrium from the left ventricle. The tricuspid valve separates the right atrium from the right ventricle. p. 405.

93. (d) The blood travels from the pulmonary vein into the left atrium. The right atrium receives blood returning from the body. p. 408.

94. (a) Storing blood for emergency use is the function of the spleen. Its second function is to destroy old red blood cells, bacteria and germs. p. 408.

95. (c) Atherosclerosis is the buildup of plaque on the arterial wall. p 408.

96. (b) Hemorrhoids is the name given to enlarged veins in the rectal area; therefore, hemorrhoidectomy is the term used to describe surgical removal of the hemorrhoids. p. 414.

97. (d) A myocardial infarction is referred to as a heart attack. p. 408.

98. (d) Leukemia is a disease characterized by rapid abnormal production of white blood cells. p. 414.

99. (c) Splenectomy means surgical excision of the spleen. The word root for spleen has only one "e" as in splen/o. pp. 411, 413.

100. (c) Thrombophlebitis is the inflammation of a vein as the result of a clot. p. 414.

101. (a) Hypertension or high blood pressure would be treated by a cardiologist. p. 413.

102. (a) An angiogram is an x-ray of the blood vessel. Angi/o is the word root for blood vessel. p. 414.

103. (b) Electrocardiography is the process of recording electrical impulses of the heart. The suffix *graphy* means process of recording, *gram* means record and *graph* means the instrument to record. pp. 414, 377.

104. (d) AIDS (Acquired Immunodeficiency Syndrome is caused by the Human Immunodeficiency Virus (HIV), which infects certain white blood cells of the body's immune system and gradually destroys the body's ability to fight infection. p. 409.

CAD - Coronary Artery Disease

CHF - Congestive Heart Failure

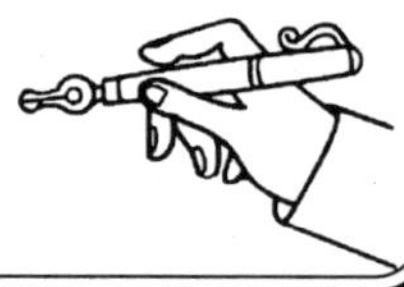

Chapter 23
Medical Terminology, Basic Human Structure, Diseases, and Disorders (Continued)

UNIT VII: The Digestive System

105. Utilization of digested food by body cells is called:

    a. metabolism
    b. digestion
    c. absorption
    d. mastication

106. Mastication occurs in the:

    a. stomach
    b. mouth
    c. rectum
    d. small intestine

107. The digestive process begins with the:

    a. food entering the stomach
    b. food entering the small intestine
    c. flow of saliva into the mouth
    d. none of the above

108. Food leaving the esophagus enters the:

    a. duodenum
    b. ascending colon
    c. stomach
    d. pyloric sphincter

109. Peristalsis is:

    a. churning of food in the stomach
    b. involuntary wave-like movements
    c. process of absorption
    d. uncontrolled coughing

110. Food leaves the stomach after how many minutes?

    a. 15
    b. 30
    c. 45
    d. 60

111. Which of the following chemically aid digestion in the stomach?

    a. intestinal juices
    b. pancreatic juices
    c. bile
    d. hydrochloric acid

112. Which of the following is *not* a portion of the small intestine?

    a. ilium
    b. jejunum
    c. duodenum
    d. ileum

113. The small intestine is how many feet in length?

    a. 5
    b. 10
    c. 15
    d. 20

114. Digestion is completed in the:

    a. small intestine
    b. large intestine
    c. rectum
    d. stomach

115. The appendix is attached to the:

    a. ascending colon
    b. cecum
    c. sigmoid
    d. rectum

116. The function of the large intestine is:

    a. elimination
    b. absorption
    c. ingestion
    d. none of the above

ANSWERS AND RATIONALE

105. (a) Metabolism is the utilization of digested foods by the body cells. p. 419.

106. (b) Mastication, the act of chewing food, takes place in the mouth. p. 419.

107. (c) The digestive process begins with the flow of saliva into the mouth from the three salivary glands: parotid, submandibular and sublingual. p. 420.

108. (c) Food leaving the esophagus enters the stomach. The function of the esophagus is simply the passage of food. p. 420.

109. (b) Peristalsis is the involuntary wave-like movement that propels food along the alimentary canal. p. 420.

110. (b) Food leaves the stomach after 30 minutes. Food continues to leave the stomach at 30-minute intervals until it is empty. p. 420.

111. (d) Hydrochloric acid and gastric juices produced by the gastric glands located in the mucous membrane lining of the stomach chemically aid in the digestion of food. p. 420.

112. (a) Ilium, a part of the pelvic bone, is not a portion of the small intestine. p. 372.

113. (d) The small intestine is 20 feet in length and is so named because it is smaller in diameter than the large intestine. The large intestine is 5 feet in length. p. 421.

114. (a) Digestion is completed in the small intestine where absorption, the transfer of digested food from the small intestine to the blood stream, takes place. p. 421.

115. (b) The appendix, which has no function, is attached to the cecum. p. 421.

116. (a) The function of the large intestine is elimination and also the absorption of water. p. 421.

NOTES:

117. Which of the following accessory organs secretes bile?

a. liver
b. gallbladder
c. pancreas
d. islets of Langerhans

118. Insulin is necessary for the metabolism of:

a. fats
b. carbohydrates
c. protein
d. fiber

119. Pancreatic juice and bile are released into the:

a. jejunum
b. ileum
c. ilium
d. duodenum

120. Which of the following procedures would *not* be used to diagnose a peptic ulcer?

a. GI series
b. gastric analysis
c. cholecystogram
d. gastroscopy

121. Gallstones lodged in the common bile duct are called:

a. cholelithiasis
b. cholecystectomy
c. choledocholithiasis
d. none of the above

122. Diverticular disease occurs:

a. on the intestinal wall
b. in the stomach lining
c. along the esophagus
d. none of the above

123. A temporary colostomy may be performed as treatment for which of the following?

a. duodenal ulcer
b. peptic ulcer
c. diverticular disease
d. cholelithiasis

124. The medical term for lesions or sores of the mucous membrane of the esophagus, stomach or duodenum is:

a. peptic ulcer
b. diverticulitis
c. gastritis
d. ulcerative colitis

125. The term which means artificial opening into the third portion of the small intestine is:

a. colostomy
b. ileostomy
c. gastrostomy
d. cheiloplasty

126. The patient was admitted to the hospital with the diagnosis of gallstones or:

a. infectious hepatitis
b. stomatitis
c. pancreatitis
d. cholelithiasis

127. Which of the following is an x-ray of the bile ducts?

a. cholecystogram
b. cholangiogram
c. upper GI series
d. abdominocentesis

128. Which of the following is an x-ray of the colon?

a. proctoscopy
b. sigmoidoscopy
c. GI series
d. barium enema

ANSWERS AND RATIONALE

117. (a) The liver secretes bile, which is stored in the gallbladder. p. 421.

118. (b) Insulin, produced by the islets of Langerhans, is necessary for the metabolism of carbohydrates. p. 421.

119. (d) Bile, which aids in the digestion of fat, and pancreatic juice are released into the duodenum. p. 421.

120. (c) A cholecystogram is used for diagnosing cholelithiasis or gallstones. p. 422.

121. (c) Choledocholithiasis is the condition of gallstones lodged in the common bile duct. p. 423.

122. (a) Diverticular disease is caused by the forming of small pouches on the intestinal wall. p. 422.

123. (c) In severe cases, a temporary colostomy may be performed as a treatment for diverticular disease. p. 422.

124. (a) Peptic ulcer is a lesion of the mucous membrane of the esophagus, stomach (gastric ulcer) or duodenum (duodenal ulcer). pp. 422, 428.

125. (b) Ileostomy is an artificial opening into the ileum, the third portion of the small intestine. p. 428.

126. (d) Cholelithiasis is the condition of gallstones. pp. 422, 428.

127. (b) Cholangiogram is an x-ray of the bile ducts. p. 428.

128. (d) Barium enema is an x-ray of the colon. p. 428.

NOTES:

129. Visual examination of the rectum is called a(an):

a. esophagoscopy
b. proctoscopy
c. sigmoidoscopy
d. gastroscopy

130. Which of the following means tumor of the liver?

a. glossoplegia
b. hepatoma
c. hepatomegaly
d. pancreatic

131. Which of the following may be performed for treatment of ulcers?

a. abdominal herniorrhaphy
b. esophagoenterostomy
c. gastrectomy, pyloroplasty, vagotomy
d. herniorrhaphy

132. Which of the following means pertaining to under the tongue?

a. stomatogastric
b. sublingual
c. glossoplegia
d. proctorrhea

Test Taking Tip: **When taking the test, take time to read the test-taking directions, then follow them carefully. Failure to do so may result in your correct answer being scored by the machine as a wrong answer. If, for example, your pencil mark is not in the exact required space, the machine may read it as an incorrect answer. Check that each question number matches the answer number. Do not hesitate to ask questions if you do not know how to proceed.**

ANSWERS AND RATIONALE

129. (b) Proctoscopy is the visual examination of the rectum. p. 429.

130. (b) Hepatoma means tumor of the liver. p. 427.

131. (c) Gastrectomy, excision of the stomach, pyloroplasty, plastic repair of the pyloric sphincter, and vagotomy, incision into the vagus nerve, are performed as a treatment for ulcers. p. 428.

132. (b) Sublingual means pertaining to under the tongue. p. 427.

NOTES:

Chapter 23
Medical Terminology, Basic Human Structure, Diseases, and Disorders (Continued)

UNIT VIII: The Respiratory System

133. External respiration is the exchange of gases between:

    a. body cells and blood in the capillaries
    b. lungs and the external environment
    c. nose and the external environment
    d. pulmonary artery and the pulmonary vein

134. During internal respiration:

    a. body cells take on oxygen
    b. body cells take on carbon dioxide
    c. lungs take on oxygen
    d. lungs give off oxygen

135. Both food and air pass through the:

    a. larynx
    b. pharynx
    c. trachea
    d. bronchi

136. The anatomical term for windpipe is:

    a. larynx
    b. pharynx
    c. bronchi
    d. trachea

137. The tubular structure located below the pharynx and connecting with the trachea is the:

    a. bronchi
    b. pharynx
    c. larynx
    d. bronchiole

138. Which of the following prevents choking?

    a. epiglottis
    b. vocal cords
    c. alveoli
    d. trachea

139. A double sac which surrounds each lung is called:

    a. alveoli
    b. pleura
    c. bronchiole
    d. none of the above

140. The exchange of gases that takes place in the lungs is between the capillaries and the:

    a. epiglottis
    b. bronchioles
    c. alveoli
    d. pleura

141. Air passes from the trachea into the:

    a. bronchioles
    b. bronchi
    c. larynx
    d. trachea

142. Collection of air or gas in the pleural cavity which results in a collapsed lung is:

    a. pulmonary embolism
    b. hemothorax
    c. pneumothorax
    d. pleuritis

ANSWERS AND RATIONALE

133. (b) External respiration is the exchange of gases between the lungs and the external environment. p. 434.

134. (a) During internal respiration body cells take on oxygen from the blood and at the same time give off carbon dioxide. p. 434.

135. (b) Both food and air pass through the throat or pharynx. p. 434.

136. (d) The trachea, which extends from the larynx to the bronchi, is the anatomical term for windpipe. p. 434.

137. (c) The larynx, also known as the voice box, connects the pharynx to the trachea and contains the vocal cords, which produce sound. p. 434.

138. (a) The epiglottis automatically covers the larynx during swallowing to prevent the food from entering the larynx. p. 434.

139. (b) The pleura is the double sac that surrounds the lung. p. 435.

140. (c) The exchange of gases takes place between the capillaries and the one-celled wall of the alveoli. p. 435.

141. (b) Air passes from the trachea into the bronchi. p. 435.

142. (c) Pneumothorax is the collection of air or gas in the pleural cavity. p. 435.

NOTES:

143. Pulmonary embolism is usually caused by a:

a. virus
b. thrombus
c. air
d. bacteria

144. Temporary stoppage of breathing is called:

a. apnea
b. asthma
c. dyspnea
d. none of the above

145. Infection of the lung is:

a. pneumothorax
b. pleuritis
c. pneumonia
d. bronchitis

146. Another term for nosebleed is:

a. rhinoplasty
b. rhinopharyngitis
c. rhinorrhagia
d. rhinorrhea

147. Surgical puncture and drainage of fluid from the chest cavity is:

a. abdominocentesis
b. thoracentesis
c. thoracotomy
d. tracheostomy

148. An artificial opening into the windpipe is a:

a. tracheostomy
b. tracheotomy
c. thoracotomy
d. thoracentesis

149. A disease characterized by destructive changes in the walls of the alveoli is:

a. pneumonia
b. emphysema
c. pleuritis
d. asthma

150. Which of the following terms is spelled incorrectly?

a. tonsillitis
b. rhinoplasty
c. tonsillectomy
d. tracheoesophageal

151. An x-ray of the bronchi and the lung is:

a. bronchitis
b. bronchogram
c. bronchoscope
d. bronchoscopy

152. Excision of the voice box is:

a. lobectomy
b. laryngectomy
c. laryngitis
d. pharyngitis

153. Which of the following is spelled incorrectly?

a. adnoiditis
b. endotracheal
c. pulmonary
d. bronchotracheal

154. Paralysis of the throat is:

a. laryngoplegia
b. pharyngoplegia
c. laryngopexy
d. pharyngopexy

143. (b) Pulmonary embolism is usually caused by a thrombus that has been dislodged from a leg vein and now blocks the pulmonary artery. p. 436.

144. (a) Apnea is the temporary stoppage of breathing. p. 438.

145. (c) Pneumonia is an inflammation or infection of the lung. p. 439.

146. (c) Rhinorrhagia is another term for nosebleed. Also called Epistaxis. p. 439.

147. (b) Thoracentesis is the surgical puncture and drainage of fluid from the chest cavity. p. 438.

148. (a) Tracheostomy is the artificial opening into the windpipe. p. 438.

149. (b) Emphysema, a degenerative disease, is characterized by destructive changes in the walls of the alveoli. p. 439.

150. (a) Tonsil has one "l" but the word root for tonsil is tonsill/o; therefore, tonsillitis has two "l"s. pp. 437, 438.

151. (b) Bronchogram is an x-ray of the bronchi and lung. p. 439.

152. (b) Laryngectomy is the excision of the voice box. p. 438.

153. (a) The correct spelling is adenoiditis. p. 438.

154. (b) Pharyngoplegia is paralysis of the throat. p. 438.

NOTES:

UNIT IX: The Urinary System and the Male Reproductive System

155. The function of the urinary system is to:

  a. produce waste material in the blood
  b. remove waste material from the blood and excrete it from the body
  c. remove waste material from the body cells
  d. none of the above

156. The basic unit of the kidney that removes waste material from the blood is called:

  a. neuron
  b. nephron
  c. renal pelvis
  d. ureter

157. The tube that extends from the kidney to the bladder is called:

  a. urethra
  b. ulna
  c. ureter
  d. urinary tube

158. The urinary bladder:

  a. produces urine
  b. adds fluid to urea
  c. provides a passageway for urine
  d. provides a container for urine

159. What percent of urine is waste material?

  a. 5%
  b. 10%
  c. 15%
  d. 20%

160. The hormone secreted by the male reproductive system is:

  a. progesterone
  b. estrogen
  c. parathormone
  d. testosterone

161. Sperm is produced in the:

  a. vas deferens
  b. urethra
  c. seminiferous tubules
  d. prostate gland

162. The epididymis is located in the:

  a. abdomen
  b. scrotum
  c. testes
  d. prostate gland

163. The prostate gland:

  a. has no function
  b. assists in the passage of urine
  c. aids in the motility of sperm
  d. aids in the production of sperm

164. The term which means "pertaining to urine" is:

  a. urination
  b. urinary
  c. urology
  d. void

ANSWERS AND RATIONALE

155. (b) The function of the urinary system, also called the excretory system, is to remove waste from the blood and excrete it from the body. p. 443.

156. (b) Over one million nephrons located in each kidney are made up of a system of arteries, capillaries, and tubes. Their function is to remove waste material from the blood. p. 443.

157. (c) The ureter, approximately 10 to 12 inches in length, extends from each kidney to the urinary bladder. It provides a passageway for urine. p. 443.

158. (d) The urinary bladder is the container for urine. p. 443.

159. (a) Approximately 5% of urine is waste material; the remainder is water. The daily amount produced by the kidney is 1500 cc. p. 444.

160. (d) Testosterone is secreted by the testicles and is responsible for the development of the male secondary sex characteristics. p. 444.

161. (c) Sperm is produced in the seminiferous tubules. p. 444.

162. (b) The epididymis is a tiny 20-inch tube located in the scrotum atop the testicle. p. 444.

163. (c) The prostate gland secretes a fluid that aids in the motility of sperm. p. 445.

164. (b) Urinary means pertaining to urine. p. 448.

NOTES:

165. The patient was admitted to the hospital with the diagnosis of "renal calculi," also called:

a. pyelonephritis
b. uremia
c. nephritis
d. nephrolithiasis

166. The term for "excision of one or both testes" is:

a. orchiectomy
b. prostatectomy
c. circumcision
d. vasectomy

167. Urethrorrhaphy means:

a. suture of a urethral tear
b. plastic repair of the urethra
c. removal of a stone
d. hemorrhage from the urethra

168. Which of the following terms is spelled incorrectly?

a. urologist
b. urology
c. ureteralgia
d. scrotem

169. Incision into the kidney to remove a stone is:

a. nephrectomy
b. nephropexy
c. nephrolithotomy
d. nephrolithiasis

170. Urine in the blood is:

a. hematuria
b. uremia
c. hydrocele
d. cystocele

171. Surgery to remove a portion of the prostate is:

a. vasectomy
b. transurethral resection
c. orchiectomy
d. laparotomy

172. A laboratory test used to determine kidney function is:

a. hemoglobin
b. urinalysis
c. blood urea nitrogen
d. hematocrit

173. Visual examination of the bladder is:

a. cystogram
b. cystoscopy
c. cystography
d. cystoscope

174. Inflammation of the bladder is:

a. nephritis
b. cystocele
c. cystitis
d. nephrolithiasis

ANSWERS AND RATIONALE

165. (d) Renal calculi and nephrolithiasis are both medical terms for kidney stones. pp. 445, 448.

166. (a) Orchiectomy means excision of one or both testes. p. 448.

167. (a) Urethrorrhaphy means suture of a urethral tear. p. 448.

168. (d) The correct spelling is scrotum. p.444.

169. (c) Nephrolithotomy is the incision into the kidney to remove a stone. p. 448.

170. (b) Uremia is urine in the blood. p. 449.

171. (b) Transurethral resection is surgery performed to remove a portion of the prostate gland through the urethra. p. 448.

172. (c) Blood urea nitrogen (BUN) is a laboratory test used to determine kidney function. p. 449.

173. (b) Cystoscopy is the visual examination of the bladder. p. 449.

174. (c) Cystitis is inflammation of the bladder. p. 448.

NOTES:

Chapter 23
Medical Terminology, Basic Human Structure, Diseases, and Disorders (Continued)

UNIT X: The Female Reproductive System

175. Which of the following is not a function of the female reproductive system?

   a. produce ovum
   b. produce hormones
   c. provide for conception
   d. excrete waste

176. The main body of the uterus is called:

   a. cervix
   b. fundus
   c. vagina
   d. none of the above

177. The female reproductive cell or ovum is produced by the:

   a. ovaries
   b. uterus
   c. fallopian tube
   d. vagina

178. Fertilization usually takes place in the:

   a. fallopian tube
   b. uterus
   c. vagina
   d. ovaries

179. Estrogen and progesterone are produced by the:

   a. ovaries
   b. fallopian tubes
   c. uterus
   d. vagina

180. The hormone "progesterone" helps in the:

   a. menstrual cycle
   b. development of female reproductive organs
   c. development of breasts
   d. preparation of the uterus for conception and pregnancy

181. The muscular tube, 3 inches in length, that connects the uterus to the outside of the body is the:

   a. urethra
   b. rectum
   c. vagina
   d. none of the above

182. The perineum is the:

   a. base of the uterus
   b. lateral portion of the buttocks
   c. area between the vaginal opening and the anus
   d. area of the pelvic floor anterior to the meatus

183. The medical term which means "without menstrual discharge" is:

   a. metrorrhagia
   b. dysmenorrhea
   c. amenorrhea
   d. metrorrhea

184. Which of the following is spelled incorrectly?

   a. gynecologist
   b. gynecology
   c. ureterovaginel
   d. uterine

175. (d) Excreting waste is not a function of the female reproductive system. p. 452.

176. (b) The main body of the uterus is called the fundus. p. 453.

177. (a) The ovum is produced by the ovaries. p. 453.

178. (a) Fertilization usually takes place in the fallopian tube. p. 453.

179. (a) Estrogen and progesterone are produced by the ovaries. p. 453.

180. (d) Progesterone helps in preparing the uterus for conception and pregnancy. p. 453.

181. (c) The vagina connects the uterus to the outside of the body. p. 453.

182. (c) The pelvic floor of both the male and female is called the perineum and the term is also used to describe the area between the vaginal opening and the anus of the female. p. 453.

183. (c) Amenorrhea means without menstrual discharge. p. 458.

184. (c) Ureterovaginal is the correct spelling. p. 457.

NOTES:

185. Hysterosalpingo-oophorectomy is the surgical removal of the:

   a. ovaries, uterus and fallopian tubes
   b. ovaries, uterus and cervix
   c. fallopian tubes, uterus and vagina
   d. ureter, ovaries and fallopian tubes

186. The surgical procedure to scrape the inner walls of the uterus is:

   a. colporrhaphy
   b. dilatation and curettage
   c. perineorrhaphy
   d. hysterectomy

187. Cervicectomy is the medical term for:

   a. inflammation of the cervix
   b. excision of the cervix
   c. incision of the cervix
   d. none of the above

188. Which of the following is spelled incorrectly?

   a. menapause
   b. menstrual
   c. vaginal
   d. menstruation

189. Surgical removal of the ovary is:

   a. oophorectomy
   b. salpingectomy
   c. salpingo-oophorectomy
   d. none of the above

190. The term which means "visual examination of the vagina" is:

   a. vaginal speculum
   b. colposcopy
   c. colposcope
   d. cervical Pap smear

191. Salpingocele means:

   a. herniation of the fallopian tube
   b. herniation of the ovary
   c. inflammation of the fallopian tube
   d. inflammation of the ovary

192. Which of the following means "pertaining to birth":

   a. natal
   b. neonatal
   c. postnatal
   d. prenatal

193. Which of the following is spelled incorrectly?

   a. obstetricion
   b. obstetrics
   c. abortion
   d. amniotic fluid

194. The medical term which means "present at birth" is:

   a. fetus
   b. congenital
   c. placenta
   d. none of the above

195. Ectopic pregnancy means:

   a. fertilized ovum implanted outside of the uterus
   b. fertilized ovum implanted inside the uterus
   c. fertilized ovum implanted in the ovary
   d. none of the above

ANSWERS AND RATIONALE

185. (a) Hysterosalpingo-oophorectomy is the surgical removal of the ovaries, uterus and fallopian tubes. p, 457.

186. (b) Dilatation and curettage is the surgical procedure to scrape the inner walls of the uterus. p. 457.

187. (b) Cervicectomy means excision of the cervix. p. 457.

188. (a) Menopause is the correct spelling. p. 457.

189. (a) Oophorectomy is the surgical removal of the ovary. p. 458.

190. (b) Colposcopy is the visual examination of the vagina and cervix. p. 458.

191. (a) Salpingocele is the herniation of the fallopian tube. p. 458.

192. (a) Natal means pertaining to birth. p. 461.

193. (a) Obstetrician is the correct spelling. p. 461.

194. (b) Congenital means present at birth. p. 461.

195. (a) Ectopic pregnancy is a fertilized ovum implanted outside of the uterus. p. 461.

NOTES:

Chapter 23
Medical Terminology, Basic Human Structure, Diseases, and Disorders (Continued)

UNIT XI: The Endocrine System

196. Which of the following is a function of the endocrine system?

    a. connection and control
    b. control and communication
    c. communication and circulation
    d. none of the above

197. Endocrine secretions go directly into the:

    a. ducts
    b. glands
    c. blood stream
    d. brain

198. Which of the following is often referred to as the "master gland"?

    a. pituitary
    b. adrenal
    c. thyroid
    d. none of the above

199. Which of the following is not produced by the anterior lobe of the pituitary gland?

    a. ADH
    b. TSH
    c. GH
    d. ACTH

200. Which of the following stimulates contraction of the uterus during childbirth?

    a. thyroxin
    b. oxytocin
    c. parathormone
    d. none of the above

201. Iodine is necessary in the body for the production of:

    a. thyroxin
    b. oxytocin
    c. antidiuretic hormone
    d. none of the above

202. The hormone necessary for the metabolism of carbohydrates is:

    a. oxytocin
    b. thyroxin
    c. insulin
    d. parathormone

203. Epinephrine is produced by which of the following glands:

    a. adrenal cortex
    b. adrenal medulla
    c. thyroid
    d. parathyroid

204. The amount of calcium in the blood is regulated by which of the following glands?

    a. parathyroid
    b. thyroid
    c. adrenal
    d. pituitary

205. Which of the following maintains metabolism of body cells?

    a. thyroxin
    b. oxytocin
    c. epinephrine
    d. norepinephrine

ANSWERS AND RATIONALE

196. (b) The function of the endocrine system is similar to that of the nervous system to communicate and to control. p. 463.

197. (c) Endocrine glands are ductless glands and do not have tubes to carry secretions to other parts of the body. The secretions go directly into the blood stream. p. 463.

198. (a) The pituitary gland is referred to as the "master gland" because it produces hormones that stimulate function of the other endocrine glands. p. 463.

199. (a) ADH is produced by the posterior lobe of the pituitary gland. pp. 463, 464.

200. (b) Oxytocin, produced by the anterior lobe of the pituitary gland, stimulates contraction of the uterus during childbirth. p. 464.

201. (a) Iodine is necessary in the body for the production of thyroxin. p. 464.

202. (c) Insulin is necessary for the metabolism of carbohydrates in the body. p. 464.

203. (b) Epinephrine is produced by the adrenal medulla. p. 464.

204. (a) Parathormone, produced by the parathyroid glands, regulates the amount of calcium in the blood. p. 464.

205. (a) Thyroxin, produced by the thyroid gland, maintains metabolism of body cells. p. 464.

NOTES:

206. Excessive insulin in the blood may cause:

   a. diabetic coma
   b. convulsions
   c. insulin shock
   d. extreme thirst

207. Fasting blood sugar is used to diagnose:

   a. diabetes mellitus
   b. diabetes insipidus
   c. Graves' disease
   d. Addison's disease

208. Which of the following terms means "disease of a gland"?

   a. adenitis
   b. adenoid
   c. adenoma
   d. adenosis

209. Which of the following is caused by lack of production of hormones by the adrenal gland?

   a. Cushing's disease
   b. diabetes mellitus
   c. diabetes insipidus
   d. Addison's disease

210. Another name for hyperthyroidism is:

   a. hypothyroidism
   b. Graves' disease
   c. Cushing's disease
   d. Addison's disease

211. A disease caused by inadequate antidiuretic hormone production is:

   a. diabetes insipidus
   b. diabetes mellitus
   c. Cushing's disease
   d. Graves' disease

ANSWERS AND RATIONALE

206. (c) Excessive insulin in the blood may cause insulin shock, whereas too much sugar in the blood may cause diabetic coma. p. 464.

207. (a) Fasting blood sugar is a laboratory test that determines the amount of sugar in the blood after fasting. It is used to diagnose diabetes mellitus. pp. 464, 217.

208. (d) Adenosis means disease of the gland. p. 466.

209. (d) Addison's disease is caused by lack of production of hormones by the adrenal glands. p. 466.

210. (b) Graves' disease is another name for hyperthyroidism. p. 464.

211. (a) Diabetes insipidus is caused by inadequate antidiuretic hormone production. p. 466.

NOTES:

SECTION VI

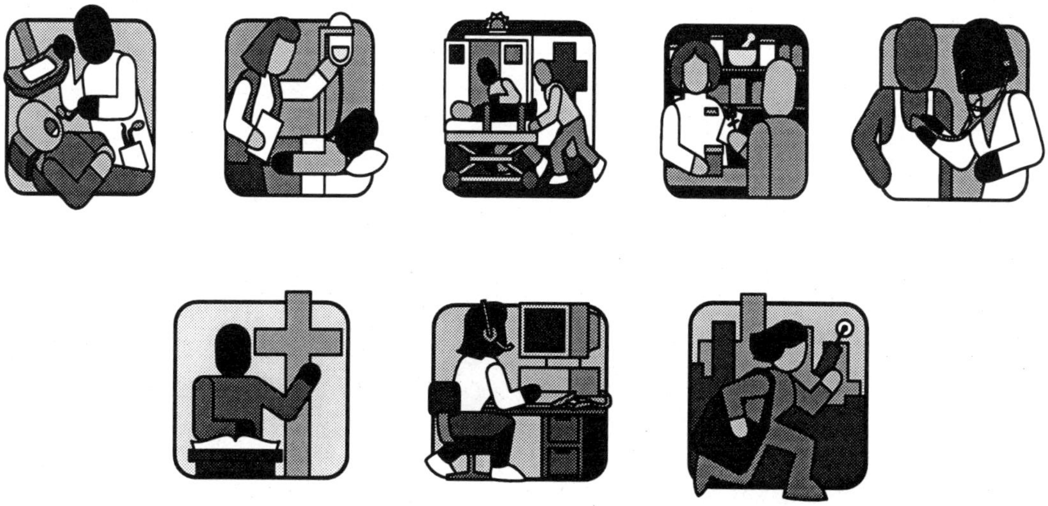

HEALTH UNIT COORDINATOR EMPLOYMENT RELATED SITUATIONS

Chapter 24
Health Unit Coordinator Employment Related Situations

The questions in this chapter cover work related situations dealing with information not covered in the textbook Health Unit Coordinating. They are intended to measure your problem solving and decision making abilities.

1. Dr. M. Hart is a cardiologist and attending physician for patient Les Breath. Dr. P. Neumon, a consulting pulmonary specialist wrote an order to transfer patient Les Breath out of CCU. To process this transfer you should (first):

   a. report the new room number to Dr. Hart's office
   b. call admitting for a bed assignment
   c. prepare the patient's chart for transfer
   d. confirm the order with Dr. Hart

2. To obtain a patient's old records from another hospital, you should:

   a. contact the patient's physician
   b. obtain the patient's consent and notify medical records
   c. obtain the patient's consent and notify the admissions clerk
   d. call Health Care Records at the other hospital

3. An order for "Quantitative Fecal Fat" would require you to:

   a. send a requisition to chemistry
   b. request a stool collection container for Quantitative Fecal Fat from the laboratory department
   c. obtain a stool specimen container for Quantitative Fecal Fat from SPD
   d. tell the nurse to obtain a stool specimen container for Quantitative Fecal Fat from the floor supply closet

4. The surgeon has written an "NPO 2400 HRS" order for a patient who is having an open reduction of right femur at 1330 tomorrow. An hour later the anesthesiologist came by to write pre op orders and ordered a "clear liquid breakfast at 0600 then NPO." You should:

   a. order the NPO 2400 hrs
   b. check with the patient's nurse
   c. order the clear liquid breakfast, then NPO
   d. call the surgeon to clarify order

5. You have repeatedly observed a young resident taking medical supplies from the nursing unit supply closet. You should:

   a. report the incidents to the nurse manager
   b. do nothing
   c. advise the resident that next time you will report him
   d. call security

6. It is 2000 and the Diagnostic Imaging Department is closed. A doctor has written an order for a "stat CT of brain to R/O brain tumor". You should:

   a. tell the nurse of the situation
   b. leave the order for next HUC
   c. ask the operator to page the CT technician on call
   d. do all other orders and wait until department opens again

ANSWERS AND RATIONALE

1. (d) The order should be confirmed with Dr. M. Hart since Dr. P. Neumon is the consulting doctor. The patient's attending doctor is Dr. A. Heart.

2. (b) The patient's consent is needed to obtain records from another hospital. Health Records will send the patient's signed consent and make the request to obtain the records from the other hospital.

3. (b) An order for a 24-72 hour specimen would require a collection container from the laboratory - it is vital that when requesting a collection container from the laboratory that you specify the test to be done so the laboratory personnel may add any additives necessary.

4. (c) Order the clear liquid breakfast, then NPO as it is the anesthesiologist's responsibility to order the pre op diet.

5. (a) Report the incidents to the nurse manager. Missing supplies are charged to the nursing unit.

6. (c) Ask operator to page the CT technician on call. There is always a technician on call for emergency situations.

NOTES:

7. A doctor has written an order for an "Echocardiogram today." The technicians are all busy and no one is in the department to take the call. You should:

   a. leave a message on department answering machine
   b. leave the order for next shift
   c. tell nurse of situation
   d. do all other orders and call later

8. A CBC was ordered on the wrong patient. The results came back with an elevated WBC. You should:

   a. place the results in the patient's (with the elevated WBC) chart
   b. order the CBC on the correct patient and discard the CBC results that were done in error
   c. call results to the doctor of the patient with the elevated WBC with the explanation that the CBC was done by mistake, then order the CBC on the correct patient.
   d. call the doctor who ordered the test and explain the situation

9. A patient is hemorrhaging, the nurse asks you to go to the blood bank to pick up the unit of blood that is ready for the patient. A doctor arrives at the same time and asks you to obtain lab results on one of his patients. You should:

   a. tell the doctor that you don't have time to wait on him/her
   b. obtain lab results for doctor then go to the blood bank
   c. ask nurse what to do
   d. advise the doctor you have an emergency and go to the blood bank

10. There is a fire in the visitors lounge which has been reported. Your reaction should be to:

   a. evacuate patients from nursing unit
   b. close all doors
   c. collect and remove all charts from nursing unit
   d. do nothing, your job is nonclinical

11. A medical student in a teaching hospital wrote orders on a newly admitted patient. The hospital policy states that medical students may not write orders. You would:

   a. page the appropriate resident to co-sign the orders
   b. call the patient's attending doctor to verify the orders
   c. transcribe the orders
   d. ask the patient's nurse to co-sign orders

12. A doctor wrote orders on a patient and forgot to sign them. It is a hospital policy that orders must be signed prior to being acted upon. You should:

   a. transcribe the orders and ask doctor to sign them the next time he/she makes rounds
   b. ask the patient's nurse to co-sign them
   c. wait to transcribe the orders until they are signed
   d. advise the patient's nurse that you are calling doctor so she/he can verify the orders and sign them

13. A doctor calls out an order to you as he/she is leaving the nursing station. You should:

   a. advise the doctor that you can not take verbal orders and ask him/her to write the order
   b. write the order as given
   c. ask the charge nurse to write the order
   d. do nothing

ANSWERS AND RATIONALE

7. (a) Leave a message on department answering machine.

8. (c) Call results to patient's doctor and then order CBC on correct patient.

9. (d) Tell the doctor you have an emergency and go to the blood bank. The doctor can call the laboratory or obtain the lab results on the computer.

10. (b) Close all doors is the fire code policy. (Be aware of fire and disaster policies)

11. (a) Page the appropriate resident to co-sign orders. (Be aware of resident's patient assignments and schedule)

12. (d) Advise the patient's nurse that you are placing a call to the doctor. The nurse can verify the orders, sign them and the doctor can sign them the next day.

13. (a) Advise the doctor that hospital policy prohibits you from taking verbal orders. Ask him/her to write the order.

NOTES:

14. A "hard copy" of an order refers to:

    a. the original written doctor's order
    b. the pharmacy copy of the orders
    c. duplicate copy of order from computer printer
    d. phone orders written by the nurse

15. A nurse calls out to you to call a code arrest on a patient that has a living will and a DNR order, you should:

    a. call the code
    b. remind the nurse of the living will
    c. call the patient's doctor
    d. refuse to call the code

16. A child is admitted to ER accompanied by a babysitter. The parents (legal guardian) can not be reached and the child needs immediate surgery. What would be done:

    a. the surgery would be delayed until parents can be reached
    b. the child would have surgery immediately without consent
    c. two doctors would sign the consent for surgery
    d. the babysitter without legal permission, would be asked to sign the consent

17. A patient tells you that the nurse assigned to him/her has been very rude. You should:

    a. report the complaint to the patient's nurse
    b. report the complaint to the nurse manager
    c. place a call to the patient's doctor
    d. do nothing, patients aren't your responsibility

18. A patient that is a known alcoholic and a frequent patient on your nursing unit, complains to you of a severe headache and you observe a difference in his speech. When you report this to this nurse, she states that "he is probably drunk." The patient's family tells you that they are very concerned, so you again report this to the nurse. The nurse tells you to stick to your job and she will do patient care. You should:

    a. call the doctor
    b. report the incident to the nurse manager
    c. do nothing - "Stick to Your Job."
    d. tell the family that you have done all you can.

19. A patient is scheduled for surgery and has signed the surgery consent. Now the patient tells you that she has concerns about pictures being taken during surgery. You should:

    a. advise the patient's nurse
    b. call the hospital photographer
    c. call the doctor
    d. tell her that pictures probably won't be taken

20. A patient has signed a consent for a hysterectomy but tells you that she is having doubts and would like a second opinion. An appropriate response would be:

    a. tell her "all patient's have second thoughts, don't worry."
    b. call surgery and cancel the hysterectomy
    c. call a priest to counsel her
    d. advise her nurse and doctor

ANSWERS AND RATIONALE

14. (c) A "hard copy" of an order refers to a computer printer.

15. (b) Remind the nurse of the living will and DNR. (Do not resuscitate order)

16. (c) Two doctors can sign a surgery consent in a life threatening emergency. The babysitter could not sign the consent unless provided with a document granting her/him legal permission to act as the child's legal guardian in an emergency by the parents.

17. (a) Report the complaint to the patient's nurse. Follow chain of command. There may have been a misunderstanding that was interpreted as rudeness.

18. (b) Report the incident to the nurse manager. The nurse manager would be the next person in the chain of command and the patient's welfare is the top priority.

19. (a) Advise the patient's nurse who would take the surgery consent back to patient to cross out permission to photograph and initial.

20. (d) Advise her nurse and doctor that the patient has concerns.

NOTES:

21. A patient has been discharged and the doctor asks you to do her a favor and keep the chart on the nursing station until tomorrow so she can finish the summary sheet. You should:

    a. do as asked and keep the chart on unit
    b. advise her that you can't do that
    c. send the chart to Health Records and tell her you forgot
    d. ask the nurse if that would be ok

22. When a patient expires you would call:

    a. only the attending doctor
    b. the chief of staff
    c. all doctors involved with the patient's care
    d. the clergy on call

23. A patient's mother has been staying with her son around the clock and tells you that she has not eaten and has no money. What would your most appropriate response be:

    a. loan her some money
    b. do nothing
    c. call social services
    d. give her some food from the unit dietary kitchen

24. You had asked for a weekend off two (2) months ago, but when the schedule comes out, you are scheduled to work. Your best solution would be to:

    a. tell the clinical manager when she/he comes by the nursing station
    b. work the weekend and forget your plans
    c. trade weekends with co-workers and don't involve staffing
    d. take a copy of the request to staffing and tell them there is an error.

25. A patient was just told by her doctor that he has terminal cancer. The patient comes to the nursing station and tells you that he is scared and does not want to die. An appropriate response would be:

    a. listen with empathy
    b. call a priest or pastor
    c. refer him to his nurse
    d. tell him to talk to his family

26. A patient tells you that her doctor told her that she has diabetes. She tells you that she is very confused about the severity of her illness and the treatment. Your best response would be to:

    a. look in the chart and answer her questions as much as possible
    b. call the diabetic nurse to talk to her
    c. tell her to wait until her doctor returns to get more information
    d. advise her that you will ask her nurse to come in to talk with her

27. You observe a visitor entering an isolation room without a gown and mask. Your best action would be to:

    a. ask the visitor if they can read signs
    b. do nothing, it's not your concern
    c. tell the nurse
    d. advise the visitor that a gown and mask has to be worn while visiting the patient

28. A consultation order is written for Dr. John Smith to see a patient regarding a ruptured disc. When obtaining a phone number from the doctor's roster, you see that there are three (3) Dr. John Smiths listed. You would:

    a. call the attending to clarify which Dr. Smith s/he meant
    b. call the Dr. Smith who is an orthopedist
    c. call the Dr. Smith who is an ophthalmologist
    d. call the Dr. Smith who is a geriatrist

ANSWERS AND RATIONALE

21. (b) Advise her that you cannot do that. Health Records have a limited time to complete discharge charts and to submit billing to insurances.

22. (c) All doctors involved with the patient's care should be notified.

23. (c) Call social services who could help her find a place to stay, if needed and follow up with other needs

24. (d) Take a copy of your request to staffing and tell them that an error was made. The request may have been overlooked. Taking the problem to the clinical manager could cause hard feelings. Follow chain of command.

25. (a) Listening with empathy is the best choice. It may be okay to suggest the other options, but just listening and caring is important because the patient chose you to share his concerns and feelings with.

26. (d) Advise her that you will ask her nurse to come in to talk with her. The patient's nurse would know the most about the diagnosis and proposed treatment. Also advise the patient to make a list of concerns and questions for her doctor.

27. (d) Advise the visitor of the isolation rules. It is part of the HUC's responsibilities to advise visitors of hospital rules.

28. (b) Call the Dr. John Smith that is an orthopedist who treats diseases or fractures of the musculoskeletal system.

NOTES:

29. You are transcribing a set of orders; one seems inappropriate to you. You should:

    a. ask another health unit coordinator what s/he thinks
    b. ask the nurse for interpretation
    c. assume the physician could not have made an error
    d. call the physician for clarification

30. You observe a coworker adding a decimal point to a medication dose on the MAR to cover an error. The medication nurse has already given the incorrect dose. You should:

    a. wait to see if the error is discovered or if any harm is done
    b. call Risk Management
    c. report the incident to the nurse manager
    d. call the patient's doctor

31. You walk into a patient's room and observe an orderly treating an elderly patient in an extremely rough manner. You should:

    a. notify the nurse manager
    b. call security
    c. advise the orderly that if you ever witness another incident, you will report it
    d. do nothing, patient care is not a HUC concern

32. A patient has signed his surgery consent. The morning of the scheduled surgery, the doctor changed the procedure to be done on the patient's order sheet. The patient has not yet been sedated. You should:

    a. change the procedure on the signed consent using white out
    b. make out a new consent with the new procedure and give it to the nurse for the patient to sign
    c. change the procedure on the signed consent using a line drawn through incorrect procedure
    d. change the procedure on the signed consent and ask doctor to initial

33. You are working on a busy pediatric unit and have been assigned a student health unit coordinator to train during their clinical rotation. The student has made numerous errors while transcribing patient orders and does not seem competent. You would:

    a. wait another week to see if the situation improves
    b. refuse to allow the student to transcribe patient's orders, but allow him/her to observe until the clinical rotation has ended
    c. advise the student's instructor (if on site) or the nurse manager right away
    d. just recheck all orders that the student transcribes, correct errors, and say nothing.

34. A hospital transport employee arrives on your nursing unit to deliver an ordered narcotic from the pharmacy. All of the RNs are busy and in patient rooms, you would:

    a. ask transport to leave the narcotic and you will have an RN sign the acceptance form later
    b. ask transport to wait for an RN to sign for the narcotic
    c. sign for the narcotic yourself
    d. ask one of the doctors to sign for the narcotic

35. You observe a coworker acting in a very strange manner and detect a smell of alcohol on his/her breath. You would:

    a. mind your business and do nothing
    b. advise the nurse manager
    c. call security and report the situation
    d. advise the co-worker to go home

ANSWERS AND RATIONALE

29. (d) Call the physician for clarification. Don't assume anything. Question orders, policies and procedures that do not seem appropriate.

30. (c) Report the incident to the nurse manager.

31. (a) Notify the nurse manager.

32. (b) A change in the procedure would require a new consent form and the patient would have to be informed of the procedure including risks and characteristics of the procedure (informed consent).

33. (c) Advise the student's instructor or the nurse manager right away.

34. (b) Ask transport to wait for an RN to sign for the narcotic. An RN must sign for a narcotic delivered to the nursing unit.

35. (b) Advise the nurse manager of the incident.

NOTES:

36. A patient on your unit is being kept alive by life support. A family member approaches you at the nurse's station to ask how you felt about removing the life support. You would:

a. advise the family member to talk to the doctor about it
b. tell the family member that you are not allowed to talk about that
c. tell the family member how you feel about life support
d. call the hospital priest

37. A co-worker has shared with you that s/he has a serious drug problem and does not plan on reporting or correcting the problem. The co-worker is in a position that could place patients at risk. You would:

a. wait to see if the co-worker will seek help
b. advise security
c. do nothing and respect the co-workers confidence
d. advise the nurse manager

38. A patient on your unit has been transferred to an ECF. After the patient has gone, you realize that you sent the original patient records rather than the copies. You would:

a. call the ECF and advise them of the error
b. call the patient's family and ask them to return the originals immediately
c. send the copies in the chart to health records and say nothing
d. call health records to report error immediately

39. When transcribing a physician's order for Ampicillin, you observe on the MAR (medication administration record) that the patient is allergic to PCN. You would:

a. transcribe the order, the doctor must know the patient's allergies
b. call the pharmacy
c. notify the doctor of the patient's allergy
d. ask the patient if h/she is allergic to Ampicillin

40. There are two charts in the chart rack with red tape marked "name alert". This would indicate that:

a. the patient's names are difficult to spell
b. the two patients are related
c. the two patients have the same last name
d. the two patients share the same doctor

41. You are working in a PICU and receive a call from one of the pediatric floor units that you are receiving a patient that just coded. All of the nurses on the unit are unable to leave their patients or are at lunch. You would:

a. page the nurse manager
b. call one of the other units to ask for help
c. tell the floor unit to hold the patient until a nurse returns from lunch
d. advise the floor unit to bring the patient and you will try to assist the doctors

42. A physician has made sexually intimidating remarks to you. You have asked him/her to stop, but h/she persists in making advances. You would:

a. avoid contact with the physician as much as possible and say nothing
b. report the situation to security
c. the next time a remark is made, slap him/her
d. report the situation to the nurse manager

43. A physician has written an order for a surgery consent. You are not sure of the spelling of the procedure. You would:

a. check the spelling on the surgery schedule
b. ask one of the nurses
c. check the spelling in the medical dictionary
d. call the doctor to clarify

36. (a) Advise the family member to discuss removing the patient from life support with the doctor.

37. (d) Advise the nurse manager. The patient's safety must come first.

38. (d) Call health records and report the error immediately.

39. (c) Notify the doctor of the patient's allergy.

40. (c) The two patients have the same last name. This is done to avoid errors in ordering tests and procedures and filing reports.

41. (a) Page the nurse manager.

42. (d) Report the situation to the nurse manager. No one has to tolerate sexual harassment.

43. (c) Check the spelling in the medical dictionary.

NOTES:

44. An order has been written to have a blood transfusion consent signed by the parent of a child going to surgery. You advise the nurse and s/he asks you to tell the parents not to leave so the consent can be signed. You would:

   a. just tell the parents to stay on the unit without any explanation
   b. advise the parents that the nurse has a form that needs to be signed and to please remain on the unit
   c. ignore the request because the parents are always there anyway
   d. advise the parents that a blood transfusion consent needs to be signed

45. When calling a code on a pediatric unit you should instruct the switchboard operator to:

   a. state "pediatric code"
   b. indicate "non adult code"
   c. call for all pediatricians to come to the unit stat
   d. not indicate that it is a "pediatric code"

46. A patient with which of the following diagnosis on a pediatric unit would need to be in isolation:

   a. RAD
   b. RSV
   c. FTT
   d. SNAT

47. Central service supply discrepancies are absorbed by the:

   a. recently discharged patients
   b. patients currently on the nursing unit
   c. central service department
   d. the individual nursing units

48. An incident report is initiated if a nurse:

   a. accidently takes the narcotic keys home with him/her
   b. goes to the hospital cafeteria with the narcotic keys
   c. leaves the nursing unit with the narcotic keys
   d. is late administering a narcotic to a patient

49. An order for a "chest PA and LAT this AM" was overlooked and discovered at 3:30 PM. You would:

   a. order the x-ray stat
   b. order the x-ray for the next day in AM
   c. do nothing as it was not your error
   d. order the x-ray ASAP and notify patient's nurse

50. The HUC on the day shift constantly leaves excess work for you to do. You have found orders that were written in the AM, when you arrive at 3:00 PM. You talked with him/her about this, but the situation has gotten worse. You should:

   a. talk to the nurse manager.
   b. refuse to transcribe orders written before noon.
   c. talk to the HUC again.
   d. do nothing, the nurse manager must be aware and you should not get involved

ANSWERS AND RATIONALE

44. (b) Advise the parents that the nurse has a form that needs to be signed and to please remain on the unit. The nurse will explain the need for the blood transfusion consent to the parent.

45. (a) State "pediatric code." A specialized pediatric code team including the pediatric intensivist will respond to a "pediatric code." (This may not apply if working in a smaller hospital that would not have pediatric specialists.)

46. (b) RSV (Respiratory Syncytial Virus) is a particular risk to patients that have lung dysfunction ie: bronchial pulmonary dysplasia, reactive airway disease, etc.

> RAD - Reactive Airway Disease
> FTT - Failure To Thrive
> SNAT - Suspended Non Accidental Trauma

47. (d) Central service supply discrepancies are absorbed by the individual nursing units.

> The HUC may be involved in recapturing central service supply discrepancies.

48. (a) An incident report is initiated if a nurse accidentally goes home with the narcotic keys. A locksmith will be called to change the narcotic cabinet lock.

49. (d) Order the x-ray ASAP and notify patient's nurse. Procedures are only ordered stat if the doctor writes an order for them to be done stat.

50. (a) Talk to the nurse manager about the problem as the patient's orders must be transcribed within a reasonable time.